mateology

The drink *beyond* a drink

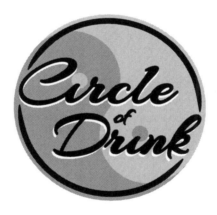

David "Mate" Askaripour

mateology

The drink *beyond* a drink

Published in the United States by:
Circle of Drink
1 Victoria Circle E. Patchogue, NY 11772
info@circleofdrink.com
www.circleofdrink.com
phone: 1 800 598 6009

Cover / Interior Design by:
Danie-J
www.danie-j.com

Second Edition, 2015
ISBN 978-0-9894944-0-3
Printed in the United States of America

Contents

INTRODUCTION

Over one hundred years ago, during the 1899 International Commercial Congress held in Philadelphia, with 38 foreign governments in attendance, the subject of yerba mate was introduced by Señor Carlos R. Santos, a Government Delegate from Paraguay:

> *Yerba maté, Paraguayan tea (ilex Paraguariensis), made from the leaves of a shrub which are pulverized or simply cured as other tea, affords a drink known by the name 'yerba maté' all through South America, where the people drinking it number 20,000,000. Maté is recommended for its hygienic, nutritious, and invigorating properties by scientific journals and notabilities, and that its general use in the United States depends solely upon its becoming more widely known is a fact beyond doubt.[1]*

It was Santos' last sentence, his prediction of yerba mate, "beyond doubt", becoming a success in the United States, that has given me the impetus to pick up where he left off and reignite interest in mate – in my home country – where it has heretofore remained prevalent only in South America. It's my sincere hope that this book acts a fulcrum, acquainting people with this plant beyond a plant; beyond a drink.

Over a century later, Santos' prediction has yet to be realized. With the early efforts of the first known mate company in the States – The Yerba Maté Tea Co. – at the turn of the twentieth-century, to the most recent efforts of Guayakí (a leading US mate company) at the turn of the twenty-first century, yerba mate still remains relatively unknown.

The time has come to expose this Miracle Herb.

My mate story begins with a trip to Argentina—finally taking the leap to learn Spanish. But it seems as though Spanish wasn't the only thing that captured my attention.

Tired, excited, anxious, and not knowing what to expect, I sat in a JFK terminal and waited for my plane to arrive. Little did I know that my eighteen-hour flight would turn into a forty-hour excursion through Mexico, Chile, then, finally, to my destination, Buenos Aires, Argentina.

Something about *Buenos Aires*, just the name alone, resonated with me. It translates as Good Air. The modern city was affectionately called "The Paris of South America." Enticing. A new language. New experiences. New faces. Many sources said "not to learn Spanish there," because of the distinct dialect of the region – spoken only in Buenos Aires and neighboring Uruguay – though, that attracted me *even more.*

I always had a knack for doing things against the grain. As far as I was concerned, my mind was made, and I bought a ticket in February. By April 2009 I was in Argentina. Who knew that I'd remain for three-years? Easily, Argentina became my second home.

The passion of the people was amazing. It's a communal, family-oriented culture. Both men and women kiss on the cheek—a required, friendly formality and sign of respect. No wonder why mate is considered "The Friendly Drink," as most Argentines can been seen sharing a gourd amongst friends and strangers alike. It's in their blood.

After two delays, heavy storms, intense turbulence, a million cat-naps, various airports, junk food, no food, sweat, and exhaustion, I arrived, depleted and blurry-eyed. Excitement overflowed as we drove into the city. Upon arrival, I threw down my bags and left to explore my new world, stitching park to park and street to street, having no clue what direction I was headed. And though the city was rustic gray and full of concrete, everything appeared resplendent and fresh. Clear sky and city pigeons abounded.

Stumbling with the few words I knew, I feebly attempted to order a vegetable pizza. The waiter, impatiently negotiating through my bastardized words and strong American accent, finally understood that all I wanted were vegetables on dough. *"Bueno!"* he said. I took my pizza and returned to the residence, a six-story renovated hotel now housing students. I lived on the top floor, in college dorm fashion —rooms packed with beds wall-to-wall. Luckily, I only had one roommate. Being twenty-five, I was one of the oldest, as the residence mostly housed young students attending local universities. There were a good share of Americans and Europeans there to learn *Castellano**, as well. Some having graduated, others on school break, and some just wanting to get away from their small towns and expand their horizons.

Seated in the kitchen, I offered the locals a slice. They weren't too interested in cheese-less pizza and after a few bites, neither was I. They looked at me like a novelty, not being accustomed to a well-dressed brown person from the USA. When I told them I was from New York, they quickly opened.

Later, while in the common room trying to be friendly and spark conversation, I noticed a few young girls forming

* Spanish dialect spoken in Argentina

4

a circle on the floor. One walked in with a spoon in a tub of what appeared to be a blob of caramel, later finding out that it was the traditional *dulce de leche*—a mixture of milk, chocolate, and sugar, heated and whipped into a syrup consistency.

"Hola...hello!" they saluted me. "Ahh...do...you...want... to...ahhh...come and join us?" "Sure, what are you girls doing?" I asked. "Do you know...ah—mate?" they asked. "Mate, what's that?" I responded with curiosity. "It's a drink we share...it's good!" "Ohh...okay sure...and what's that in the bucket?" "This is...ah...*dulce de leche*...it's good...here eat some!" while practically shoving the spoon down my mouth. "Not bad...very good," thanking them. "Here you drink now..." and so began my journey with mate.

I clasped the gourd with both hands and sheepishly sipped from this weird metal straw that brought up hot, bitter tea to my mouth. I had to force it down and try to mask my difficulty swallowing the scolding liquid, rolling down my throat like molten lead. I was a mate virgin no more.

"Do you like the mate?" another asked. "Yeah... yeahhh I do...very good. *Muy bueno.*" "Ahh...you speak castellano...? *muy bien, muy bien...*" they responded with cheer and wide smiles. "Noo, I'm actually here to learn. I know a few words, but almost nothing," I responded. "It's easy, you learn fast.

I help you!"

We all spent the next few hours eating snacks, sipping mate, and getting to know one another in Argentine fashion of good conversation, laughs, and openness. They were all so kind, patiently augmenting words to my measly vocabulary. Outstandingly warm people. I thought to myself "wow... what a nice little experience I'm having. It's only the first day, and I'm here sitting with people who were strangers only minutes ago, now sharing one straw to slurp a strange tea concoction, in harmony and sympathy with one another." I'm not sure if such an event could've taken place in New York.

I guess that's just how things work out.

Why was it that I decided on Argentina instead of Mexico? What urge nudged me to South America? What was the inkling towards alternative health in 2004, as I started to study green tea, now mate? Who were those people on the streets of Manhattan who continued to ask for directions in Spanish, sparking my desire to learn the language? Who was that girl that I met my first week in Argentina and had passionately convinced me to stick around when my classes were completed three-months later? What factors were behind becoming strongly steeped in the culture, language, food, and idiosyncrasies of this foreign land? Why did I decide to buy a gourd and bombilla? Why did JC give me that first bag of yerba? Why did I make that first youtube video explaining what mate meant to me, back in April 2010 while visiting NY? Where did these forces arise from? I don't know, but I'm here now. And mate is by my side. Our paths have met – mate's and mine – and the work we have to do together, having kindled long before we met, I feel has only just begun.

Sound dramatic? Perhaps there is a drama at play. That's the thing about mate—it's the most animated drink I've ever encountered. It's alive! It's something that seeps through the gourd and wafts out; something that isn't liquid or steam or herb. Alien substance? Is it from Earth? I like to think of it as *magic*. The indigenous peoples referred to mate as "The Drink of the Gods" and has been said to have been handed down by the God of Friendship. They prayed to their Mate God, *Caá Yará*, for their beloved plant to always grow.

I've always thought of a myth as a way to tell a truth in something made up. A way to weave lessons into a story once imagined by wise elders sitting around a fire, faithfully extolling guidance on the young. Perhaps this is how, long ago, friendship was infused into each leaf of *Ilex Paraguariensis,* what we now call Yerba Mate. Maybe it was the tears of united friends that, after years apart, found one another while standing around a mate shrub deep in the forests of Paraguay—and it was then that the mate plant, seeing this beautiful display of affection, connection, and love, cried its own tears and watered itself that evening, instructing each of its cells to forever forge friendships between whosoever drunk its leaves.

Mate, in its essence, is more than just a plant or drink or herb, but a *lifestyle*. A symbol that represents unity among everyone that sits to drink and speak whatever comes to mind. What Argentines, Uruguayans, Paraguayans, and Brazilians have been doing for centuries, passed on from generation to generation, is something, now more than ever, we North Americans can use.

A binder to bandage the mind-frying hustle and bustle of a Starbucks-paced, in and out, 1-2-3-coffee-meeting society. I think the Pacific Northwest of the United States has something going with their quaint, local coffee and tea shops catering to their fellow community members in an unpretentious, homely way.

I was intimately able to observe this sharp contrast between speeds of life while living in one of the most remote places in Northern California—Arcata, Humboldt County, population 17,000. The smallest town I've lived in. I was confused when a lady, having just left the grocery store with bags in hand, stopped to gladly offer me organic fruit juice. I cracked the bottle open and she said "go ahead, you look thirsty...take a sip." After a few sips, she took a few sips herself – after I, a total stranger had sipped it – and wished me farewell.

You have to understand that these random acts of sharing rarely happen in New York, and I'd imagine for the greater part of the States. In Argentina, seeing people share the same straw – the mate *bombilla* – touched me. Barriers were immediately disassembled in a slurp! It symbolized acceptance for the unknown and said, confidently, "I trust you."

Perhaps mate, or the fundamental traditions of it, aren't so foreign to us as we may think. As a young teen, some of my fondest memories were of myself, walking around, cruising the neighborhood, or sitting on my skateboard behind CVS or Walgreens, where we spent hours learning new tricks, passing around a joint, or sipping Old English 40s pretending to be *Boys in the Hood*. As we passed the joint, one tacitly knew that what was happening was more than just "getting buzzed," but coming together – *being together!* – and sharing ourselves with one another. Connecting. Telling our stories. Laughing at the most mundane things that had us rolling on the pavement in pain. Talking about the girls we've kissed or are *trying* to kiss. Discussing the latest graffiti artists, breakdancing moves, or repeating the hottest lyrics from *Wu Tang, The Fugees, Nirvana, Nas,* and *The Smashing Pumpkins.*

The joint, now more than a joint, became the symbol of this unspoken ritual that bonded us in the same way that wine has been called "the social lubricant," or the few cigarettes that co-workers share on a break while unburdening the daily stress of the demanding 9-to-5.

So mate isn't so different after all. But at the same time, it is *very* different. When we put aside the actual object of mate and reinstate the symbol, we see how the medium of sharing – whether it's with wine, marijuana, or mate – is the same. And it's this precise detail that seduced me to write this book and share my story. The story of an herb that has changed my life. I think that mate has a lot to offer. It's another conductor of friendship that is as foreign to the typical American now as computers were to us in the early '80s. Now look, everyone has a computer, facebook account, and an iPhone. Why? Because they just work. And so does mate—*it just works!*

Amargo is the word for bitter in castellano. Mate, being naturally bittersweet, more bitter than sweet, is often distasteful to the average American palate. We've been force-fed sweet things from infancy and have become addicted to sugar-riddled garbage that we dare call food.

10

The Mate Gods, as if acting as a Zen Master not immediately accepting the student, makes the prospective drinker go through a series of tests and challenges before allowed to experience the *true* lessons—before She shows Her magic to us.

People first need to get past the bitter taste and build a relationship with the herb before immaturely casting it off as "too bitter" and "what is this nasty stuff?" I like to imagine that people who are able to drink and enjoy bitter things, usually have more advanced and evolved minds.

I'm not saying that if you don't smoke cigars, drink espresso, and like your whisky neat, that you aren't eligible to drink mate, but only that if you take the time to adjust and adapt to mate – to let mate *readjust* you – then you'll reap the bountiful rewards. Such is the case with all amazing things in life.

How many of us *honestly* enjoyed that first sip of beer? When I was around seven or eight, my uncle convinced my dad to let me have a sip. I thought how bitter and awful tasting it was.

"You see...he doesn't really want to drink it," my uncle jeered my dad. Years later, after a friend and I stole a few beers, I tried my hand again—this time drinking an entire can. Still far from tasting great, something was different this time. Minutes after finishing, I began to feel a bit weird and slightly dizzy. Then, after adjusting, this altered, curious state began to feel interesting, then good. Giggling, I walked around our neighborhood woods feeling wonderfully buzzed. As I matured, I began to drink beer and alcohol more often and grew to enjoy not only its acquired taste, but its ability to help me "let go," albeit in a clumsy way.

Mate is an acquired taste, for sure. When I took that first sip in April 2009, I wasn't sold. Even with a palate partial to bitter things, it didn't take. I simply thought of it as *just another tea.* But as time passed, I was invited to sit in more and more circles: people gathering together to share mate over good conversation. I began to bloom and rise to mate, as if those first few sips had planted seeds that were slowly maturing and waiting to break through at the right moment.

Mate is mysterious like that. It doesn't show its true colors on the first date. You have to entertain her over and over before you gain her respect and confidence. When she feels like she can trust you, *then* she'll invite you into her house and show you a grand time. A time that you'll never forget. It won't be a one-nighter, but a lifetime of pleasure and comfort.

Most people feel "something" after a few minutes of drinking mate. This something is often described as a buzz or feeling of euphoria and alertness—others will leave it, unable to accurately describe its soothing effects, as "I feel different." I think that this has, initially, mostly to do with the new drinker not being accustomed to the stimulating and nutrifying effects of mate—a creative cocktail of excitatory and relaxing compounds also found in tea, coffee, and chocolate, but uniquely grouped in mate, not found in any other plant. The body is rebooting, and during this phase, you may feel jittery and overly-stimulated. However, once the mate uploads her software into your system, you come back sharper than before.

Theobromine, found in chocolate; caffeine, found in coffee; and theophylline, found in tea – and arguably, but now sufficiently debunked, a new stimulant called "mateine" – are all identified in mate, adding to its extraordinary and paradoxical ability to both stimulate and relax the body simultaneously.

This uncopied combination of chemicals makes for a special drink that's uplifting, energizing, and clarifying. You don't get the jitters as with coffee, but a gentle buzz that's sustainable throughout the day and slow releasing. You get the same calm and cooling effect as tea, along with the euphoria of chocolate—similar to the effects from the raw chocolate bean known as cacao. This is usually what the new drinker is describing as a "high" within those first sips. She may not know what's taking place, but simply that a new feeling of comfort and harmony has arisen like sun cutting through fog. Creative clarity. The mind is suddenly cleared and the body becomes relaxed and agile, yet remaining active and strong. Intelligent herb.

Coffee is the bully that's strong and can beat up all the weaker kids, but goes home every night exhausted, tired, and spent from all the effort and leaked energy. Mate is the supple child who waits, observes, and remains calm in the face of danger—he's always strong and sharp, never overexerting energy; only thinking when thinking is called for; acting only when acting is called for; and releases energy only if need be.

Each drinker will feel this sense of newfound energy and power, but I don't consider this the magic of mate, or at least not entirely. Though companies will lean towards marketing these aforementioned psychophysical benefits, they are only the face of mate, not the heart.

The best way I can describe mate's effect is as a *creative clarity*. Mate is the windshield wiper of the mind, clearing away obscurities to see beyond the limits of your ego. That's why mate is always associated with being around friends and talking about interesting things that not only benefit *you*, but the group. We affect the plant as much as it effects us. A symbiotic relationship. The mate speaks to us; speaks through us; and we speak to it. This is the magic of mate that goes beyond the physical sensations that indelibly affect our bodies and activate our minds.

Mate, containing healthy doses of potassium and magnesium, plays on the heart. The word heart also can spell the word earth. The heart is the gateway to the soul and it's represented energetically, not by the color red, but green; green like the mate leaves. Mate will not only help protect your heart physiologically, but also on a psychic level.

The heart is the body's greatest oscillator of blood and energy. Electromagnetically, we use it to connect to those we're around, positively or negatively. Mate's positive effects on the heart not only keep us healthy within, but also externally.

Mate is the best of coffee, tea, and chocolate, because it embodies the magic of all three plants—remember, chocolate comes from the cacao plant, which was considered the "Food of the Gods" by the Ancients. Is it any surprise that mate is called "The Drink of the Gods"?

We know that the Guaraní Tribe of Paraná have been drinking it as of the sixteenth-century, when the European imperialists noticed the natives consuming it. It's safe to say that it was being drunk long before that. But how is mate perceived in modern time?

There have been studies by Sloan Kettering that suspect mate being responsible for certain types of throat cancers, but there are dozens of articles from reputable sources that will present evidence against that claim.

Many believe that the cancer has more to do with the extremely high temperature of water[2-3] – thermal carcinogenesis – mutating the lining of the throat, increasing its exposure to cancerous formation (esophagitis). Some scientists suggest that methods in which mate is dried produce carcinogens. None of the research has been conclusive. Even the mate naysayers must admit how powerful and healthy mate is for the body. It's packed with amino acids, B vitamins, minerals, antioxidants, and nutrients—in concentrations not found in any other plant. Mate has significantly more antioxidants than both green and black tea.

Knowing that the Guaraní have been ritualistically consuming this plant for at least hundreds of years, probably thousands, is a reliable indicator of its potency.

What mate does to the nervous system is on par with what any master masseuse does to the tight and knotty muscles. It invigorates the mind, body, and spirit like no other drink can. It nimbles thought. Coffee, tea, guayusa, and the likes bow at the throne of mate's majesty.

The *prana,* or life force, within mate – also residing in all lifeforms throughout the cosmos – responsible for any intelligence and vitality of the organism – is of such a high vibration that anyone whosoever drinks it, will automatically elevate to a higher vibratory frequency. The herb doesn't just act on the physical, but the mental and spiritual faculties as well.

Mate's roots may begin in the soil, but they also set within the body of the drinker; the nervous system now being the new soil or conduit to continue its intelligence and magical restorative and creative powers. Each sip expands consciousness.

In Paraguay, after Jesuit priests first began to commercially cultivate mate, discovering the secret method for softening the hard seeds through birds' digestive tracts, it quickly became the drink for the rich and wealthy, while maintaining its dominant presence among the common man.

By the early 1900s an estimated 15 to 20 million people in South America were consuming it daily. And though efforts were being made to commercialize the drink in the United States, most notably by The Yerba Maté Tea Co. – with supporting beneficial health reports from leading scientists, chemists, and travelers who partook in the mate experience while abroad – mate never gained traction in North America. In Germany, France, and England mate was more commonly drunk.

Within well-to-do homes of settlers and affluent natives of South America, mate was, at times, presented like a finely aged wine in a high-end restaurant. The servant, after preparing the mate with the right amount of sugar (optional), milk (optional), hot water, and yerba, would take a sip to test its quality before presenting it to the head of the house sitting before his guests. The master would then take a sip to see if the mate met the measure of quality; if he approved, the servant would then add more hot water from the kettle and the master would drink the first gourd before refilling and passing it on to his guests.

It's not surprising to see mate being revered in this fashion. The Indians of South America treated cacao, raw chocolate nuts, as gold, and at times used it as currency. Mate has also been used as currency, acting as paychecks and bartering items. Here we see mate taking on a similar level of respect and homage to its immense healing and uplifting powers. The herb just makes you feel good. And anything that makes you feel good, is priceless.

It's ability to curb hunger was of immense value to the indigenous, whom at times went days without food; the Jesuits wondered how it was possible to maintain such endurance and stamina without food, and soon enough, through keen observation – now being an obvious fact – realized it was the mate sustaining them.

During the War of Triple Alliance (Paraguayan War), between Argentina, Uruguay, and Brazil against Paraguay's uprise to increase its influence over South America, the Brazilian Army, in the absence of food rations, exclusively drunk mate for three-weeks.[4] Gauchos, cowboys of the time, would carry a sack of mate to prepare during breaks between long rides.

Westerners who fortunately partook in these rituals, had the unique vantage point of experiencing the power of mate firsthand, as they also drunk from the same gourds with the locals. These men were later responsible for helping to bring mate North, urging Europeans and North Americans to try this mysterious herb that soothed and calmed the nerves.

Seeing how infrequent and rare alcoholism was in South America, mate was deemed a powerful temperance drink for the United States. "Cheers but does not inebriate" was one such slogan presenting the – what some refer to as "a high" – uplifting quality of mate without any negative side effects of aggression, loss of memory, or blacking out, which go hand-in-hand with alcohol consumption.

Rev. Dr. J. A. Zahm, C.S.C., Ph. D., having no financial interest in mate, while experiencing it in South America as not only a Reverend but esteemed Doctor, wrote the following in his paper "Through South America's Southland":

> *This kind of mate is put up in small tin cans, and I am greatly surprised that it has not yet been introduced into the United States. I am convinced it would, as soon as known, become immensely popular. It is always ready for use and easily served. Besides this it has all the virtues of tea and coffee and none of their deleterious qualities...it is the most invigorating beverage imaginable and leaves no disagreeable after-effects. For use in hospitals it is invaluable. As a temperance drink it is nonpareil. It has preserved a large part of South America from the debasing evils of alcoholism, and I can conceive of no more powerful aid to the cause of temperance in our country than the popularizing of a beverage that has proved so efficacious among millions of people in our sister continent.[5]*

As I sit here typing, a hot thermos and packed gourd to each side, I take some pleasure in knowing that perhaps I'm the only one in my town sipping the bittersweet leaves of yerba mate. Home in New York with Argentina once again on my horizon, soon I'll be in a sea of mate drinkers in the lively city of Buenos Aires, where I've been living intermittently for close to three-years.

To see mate penetrate geography, culture, race, economic status, religion, and sex is something that I will always be in awe of and, at once, never fully comprehend. Fair enough.

Perhaps there's something to be said as to why mate hasn't ignited the globe, despite being the most nutritious herb on the planet. Have you ever seen a mate commercial? Maybe it's the subtle grace of the herb, being immensely strong, yet gentle—moving slowly, but surely.

As I've said earlier, mate, as with any other plant, contains its own intelligence. Like a signature, mate, too, has an imprint on the world. It's not as hurried as coffee nor as calm as tea. It takes its own time and travels at its own pace. Starting in South America, one day it'll decide to also lay deep roots in Europe, Africa, Asia, and North America.

Currently, notwithstanding the commercial efforts once tried in the 1900s and now again as of the late 1990s, mate still remains as infinitely wise and inconspicuous as the Taoist Monk: we know that he lives in seclusion down yonder on the hillside, but we never see his face. We feel his eminence, but will not see him in the market.

Saludos, Dave Mate
December 2011 Long Island, NY

Chapter 1

What is Mateology?

Mateology is the holographic, multi-dimensional, ever-expanding nature of yerba mate. Just as the mind and body are one inseparable unity, though consisting of their respective parts, so is mate inextricably woven between itself and those that partake in drinking this ancient herb.

Mate isn't merely a *drink*, or a "tea," as it's often labeled, but an *experience;* a lifestyle; a way of communicating not only with yourself, but other mate drinkers – the satellite herb, connecting and receiving – broadcasting friendship with every sip; every fresh gourd; every warming of the kettle; every conversation; every musing; every gaze into the eyes of those with whom you share.

Mate is a manifestation – an herbal conductor of openness and friendship – that has appeared on Earth, here with us, instructing in myriad ways. Naturally showing us how to press pause on hectic society life, and press play on connecting with our fellow brothers and sisters.

Mateology can be thought of, or rather *experienced as,* the unifying fabric that spans across the unfathomable ocean of what mate means to you; how mate affects your life; the bonds that are formed through the relationship that you have with mate; and all the untold, ineffable, holy manifestations that arise from the fertile ground in which mate flourishes— from the soils of Argentina, Paraguay, and Brazil, to the hearts and homes across our globe.

Mate propagates love in every circle, or ceremony, it's shared in. Each of us will have our own unique mateology, and that's the beauty of it. Though unique, it's all connected.

Just as the neuropeptides of the brain far expand the confines of the single brain organ and enter the entire body, acting as molecular transmitters, sharing biological information, so mate works: our individual relationship with mate is but a seed in an infinitely expanding field of growth, reverberating and sending up new shoots throughout the universe. Each *Matero** sends down roots to be grown into and forever fused with *all* Materos. Mate drinkers know this inherently and easily.

We are One body, here, together. You have a body, but are also no-body. Which is to say, that you are far greater and more powerful than you may think. Mate reveals that you are not localized to any single point in time and space.

* Yerba mate enthusiast.

23

Mate has pulled me through time and space, opening a world that I had never imagined. Revealing the ridiculousness of the general acceptance of temporal time and limited space. How can my relationship with you be quantified, measured, compartmentalized, and divided? Yet, isn't that the the very basis of modern society? We've become mechanized and overly structured in such a soft, fluid, beautiful world. Plastic flowers trying to live forever as we chase through life like a marathon, constantly competing instead of cooperating.

In the short essay, *Basis of Leisure,* renowned philosopher Josef Pieper brilliantly frames leisure not as something to be avoided or looked down upon, but an absolutely necessary element for the development of the individual and the making of a healthy culture.

Let us not confuse *leisure* with lazy. To practice leisure is to fall back into yourself, taking time to sigh out false and breath in truth; to contemplate and meditate; to tap into the unfathomable depth of your inner cosmos. Did not the Shamans, Philosophers, Poets, and the greatest scientific minds of our history take time to enjoy life? "*Sincerely,* not seriously" as philosopher Alan Watts often said. To reflect on this beautiful flow we call life.

Some understood the inviolable law of Nature: to be just as much interested, *if not more*, in the development of *myself,* as I am with the outer world. Understanding that there is really only an illusion, *maya*, that divides our thinking into believing that what is outside is not also inside, and what is inside is not also outside. Mate is one of the greatest solvents for dissolving this myopia.

As I've written in the introduction, mate is no greater than any other medium of sharing—be it tea, a joint, or a round of beers. Sure, each have their own resonance and attached, quote unquote, acceptances and social standings within any given society, but fundamentally they all achieve the same end. The differences are what we energize each medium with—what spiritual, social, and accepted colors we paint them.

Mate is something that has been deeply imbued with *sharing energy;* it resonates with connecting powers. It's vibrating at such a high spiritual frequency and so richly charged with a primordial vital force behind all consciousness, *prana,* that one cannot help but be mesmerized by its alluring ability to melt socially constructed barriers such as: race, religion, gender, sexuality, and socioeconomic status. It dissolves them into a rich amalgam of friendship and unity.

It is no surprise that mate also supplies immense healing and life rejuvenating powers. The twenty-first century pharmacology of mate is still in its infancy stages, but researchers such as University of Illinois, Associate Professor of Food Chemical and Toxicology, Elvira de Mejia, have found caffeine derivatives in mate to be effective in successfully destroying colon cancer cells, published in *Molecular Nutrition & Food Research.*[1]

The *Guaraní* have been using mate as a basis for most of their medicines since untold times, long before the Spanish and Portuguese entered their territories.[2]

The research on mate's health properties continue to erupt into the mainstream, with mentions on the popular health show, *Dr. Oz.*[3] I openly embrace the science of mate and look forward to its growing pharmacopeia.

So it is in this light, that Mateology has manifested within me. I was originally going to name this book "More than a Drink," but decided that such a name would do this work no justice. It would be to overstate the simple fact.

Chapter 2

Creative Clarity

A mate circle is one of the most creative events taking place on Earth. Sitting around your friends, or anyone, with a mate, you're right away creating a connection.

This isn't just some whimsical, romanticized event. It's heart-to-heart connection. It's *imaginal,*[1] meaning that your subjective experience manifested throughout the circle will, in fact, affect everyone else in the circle—hopefully in a positive manner. Likewise, the collective thoughts that inevitably manifest within the circle will penetrate the creatively-steeped minds of the Whole.

Everyone is creating; whether it be within their own thoughts, or the thoughts and musings shared throughout the circle. A creative platform of the highest degree is established and the podium is equally shared.

There's a popular phrase in castellano: *"La bombilla no es un micrófono,"* the bombilla isn't a microphone, so pass it on, is the idea. But in many ways, during a circle, the microphone *is* your bombilla; your guests become an audience; as for any praise, it's not needed; that'll be felt simply by sitting within the circle, as the creative resonance reverbs throughout the ceremony and further beyond, throughout the building—and further, beyond the Earth; beyond the Cosmos.

A bond has formed amongst you and the circle, and no matter if not even a word is spoken, a conversation is taking place. Doctors say that our hearts are 60% neurons,[2] the same cells of the brain. This doesn't surprise me.

For millennia, the Ancients knew that truth passes through the heart, not (only) the mind. The mind is the home for the ego – for the personality, the *persona*, or mask, we've created – the thing that we constantly *think* we are, but never are. We think it, because we create a "body image"[3] for ourselves: we believe that we are only a person stuck inside a biological body bag that is born then grows old and dies because we feel pain. I know that we are more than a body, and that the mind isn't localized to our physical.

The mate server, in a way, becomes a guide, or guru, for those that he or she is serving. The act of preparing the mate, then serving it, is a lesson in and of itself, being imparted on to the Whole. It's a great act of humility to invite someone to your home, then serve them over and over again.

The best mate servers are the ones that drop the lowest. The ones that aren't afraid to, if only for *one hour*, expose themselves. I don't think that being a man or woman is

28

so much about the ability to earn money or have a title or rank in some school or job, as it's determined by the *inner work* that has either been carried out or restrained. To show love is tremendous work. To be horrible to others is easy, lower work.

Serving mate is a practice of high caliber. Each time you initiate a circle, is a chance to not only serve a good mate, but an opportunity to boil out the impurities of your spirit and mind—to invite the All to sit amongst you, in silence. It may not be seen, but always felt. Mate is a symbol of maturity and coming to age.

In LaBerge's seminal book, *Exploring the World of Lucid Dreaming*, I read of one German scientist, Hermann Helmholtz.[4] He describes three stages of creativity as: saturation, incubation, and illumination. The saturation phase is when we begin to approach a problem: studying it, poking at it, having a few goes at it, playing with it, and immersing yourself in the intricacies and subtleties. You may be studying a solution on how to overcome your fear of heights. In this stage, you're considering and researching possible solutions.

The next stage is the incubation of the problem, when you stop actively trying to solve anything. Some people may *walk it off* in the park; others take naps to inadvertently tackle the problem in the subtle, dream world. This is the stage of fermentation and gestation of the problem. It's stirring like a kettle of mate water, slowly reaching its temperature. The problem is totally forgotten on a conscious level, but continues to percolate in the subconscious.

The last phase is illumination. This is the time when you suddenly say "yes, I got it!" The moment when you're abruptly awoken and madly jotting down solutions to the problem you've been working on, have let go of momentarily, and now coming to that "Eureka!" The moment you've been waiting for. You've turned the light on in a dark place. Neural nets have connected and a bridge has forged the once unknown to the known.

Mate prepares the mind for illumination of ideas. I call it "creative clarity." Mate puts your mind in a state of meditation, or what the Taoist call "no-mind." When the mind is out of the way, there's space—room to grow. Room for the new.

Only out of nothing can we ever have something. Mate clears the slate, *tabula rasa,* and reboots your mental drive. Maybe it's a result of the magnesium or B vitamins that mate abounds with, inciting soothing and clearing sensations.

Or perhaps it's the unique chemical cocktail of alkaloids: theobromine, caffeine, and theophylline. Chocolate enthusiasts know that it's the theobromine that helps you feel happy.

Or maybe it's beyond all these parts, yet including them, as a result of the greater, more subtle, *pranic* energy, or magic, if you will, that not only constitutes mate, but *IS* mate.

When each person grabs hold of the mate and begins to sip this ancient elixir, a gateway is opened into the soul. A place where I do not believe the mind can enter, or at least not completely. We may reflect and contemplate, but yet, I am still not convinced that these activities are the fodder of ideas and creativity. To be whole, healthy, or holy – words from the same source – one needs to be empty or hollow – like bamboo.

This contradicts the western thought of: those that work the hardest, think the hardest, do *anything* the hardest, will be most handsomely rewarded. In some ways that holds true. But to what end? What shall be your reward. Will it be the measure of money you've accumulated? Will it be the amount of people whom can remember your name, or look up to you with starry-glazed eyes?

Or will your reward simply be the *knowing* that you've done the work. What work? *Your work.* Don't you know that you chose to come here, to carry out your mission. Don't you know that your every dream is just as real as your every waking moment. So pay attention. Literally, be attentive and aware to every single moment: in your dream body or physical, for you are, fundamentally, neither and both.

Mate is a spaceship that takes you out of your limited personality. You and the other Materos board together and shoot straight out of societal orbit, into the cosmos. This shuttle inevitably malfunctions because it's fueled with remnants of your egos and lingering thoughts—burned away in the disintegration of the travel.

Each person perishes and reintegrates into the Whole of existence. No persons remain, just One. Unity. Wholeness. Tao. Hollowness. And it is in the space of no-thing, that all creativity is born. Each sip a death of your ego and rebirth of your true essence.

Slurp!

Chapter 3

Mate Circles

Tea drinking is best suited to a veranda or a quiet room; near a
bright window with a table of gnarled wood; in a monk's hut or a
Daoist hall; under moonlight silhouetted by bamboo thickets with
wind blowing through the pine trees; while sitting at a banquet and
reciting poetry; while discussing matters and reading scrolls.[1]

- THE ANCIENT ART OF TEA

A mate circle is the polar opposite of being in a club. Instead
of trying to impress or get someone's attention with your
best dance moves and new clothing, the mate circle naturally
equalizes everything, allowing a moment of "just being."

We move forward up the corporate ladder, not by our
hard work, but by *trying hard to impress* the right people. We
try, we try, we try, we try some more. If trying doesn't work,
we use money to skip the hurdles. This is common.

Mate is objective-less. It's the solvent that cuts through
this game; all games. If you ask me for the truth, I don't
believe in *trying* anything. To try, is to lie. To be, is true. "Sit
still and you will know that I am God."

33

When I go to the clubs, I reaffirm what I already know. I am never impressed by the display of barbarism, excessiveness, manipulation, and exhibition of male-dominated control—a microcosm of the grander society.

Each gourd brings me closer to the simplicity of mate. You may think of me as romantic and *loco,* so be it. "More than fame, than money, than wishes, give me truth!—'Give me mate!' "

Mate is the most calming and activating drink in the world. It's for relaxing as well as jumpstarting your day. It'll do what needs to be done. An adaptogen of the highest caliber.

When drunk amongst a group, it'll do its magic, connecting minds and hearts. Telepathy will become the norm. A mind? Forget it. Your heart will now do all the communicating as the mind downshifts a gear. Each person will ooze and melt into the next. Each individual will be murdered by the mate and resurrected as a God. The hanging caterpillars will hear the resounding *slurrrp slurrpp* of the bombilla and immediately explode from their slumbering cocoons in rapture and vigor, transform like Hulk and take flight, lingering above your heads – intoxicated – basking in the fresh sweet scent of the yerba. A sparrow will alight the brim of your gourd – each person will not be surprised, but accepting – as it then plucks a *palo* and brings it back to its nest. Three-years later, a squirrel will rip it apart,

34

inadvertently incorporating it into his nest, high above the pines. Your thoughts will transpose with each Matero and suddenly you'll become as sensitive as a girl, thinking about "what was it that upset mom earlier this morning?" And each girl will think manly thoughts and take on a sudden interest in speed, strength, and bravado. The left hemisphere will play hop scotch with the right. The right will dare the left to dream. The left will double dare the right to calculate. Then they'll combine and call their child *Matesync.*

Learning how to prepare mate pales in comparison to learning how to *infuse yourself* into the mate.

You first must understand the *experience* of mate, the purpose of why we come together—then your mind, body, heart, and spirit will be in the best place to make the mate; to infuse it with your entire Self. Seeds only germinate under the right conditions.

Each sip is sacred.

• • •

When I die fill my grave with yerba. Place me in naked. Let it rain and allow the mate to seep deeply into my shell. I'll sit on my tomb in ethereal form and project back into my physical just to take a sip, then fly off to the Fifth Dimension to float in full lotus with the Mate Gods, learning about the ancient force that fuels mate's magic. Like the sleeping Kundalini, they'll show me how those special humans awaken and rise mate's true magic up to their crown chakra, through the sushumna bombilla, with the explosion of the thousand-petaled ilex. A cloud of polvo will fill the air with resplendent scintillas, irradiating brilliant light. After my 360 degree life review, I'll apply to be resurrected in Misiones and sprout not through the womb, but through the soil, to be drunk for a thousand-years.

Not long ago I explained mate to someone. I cryptically responded: "It has theobromine from chocolate, theophylline from tea, and caffeine from coffee, which makes it unique."

I felt remiss after seeing her puzzled face, as if she had said: "what the heck did you just say…?" The better answer would have been "mate is a drink that brings people together."

There's an alchemy at play with mate. Barriers are being pulverized into the makings of golden moments. From tension and stress, calm and relax are the new elements. Race distinctions and social statuses are quickly melted into the unmovable, yet flexible, brass of unity. Mate is the medicine of the millennia. The circle represents a social caldron of healing.

How *busy* our lives are becoming! We're stuck in boxes

all day, sequentially paging through life like leaves in a book —school, college, work, work, work. How often do we take time to contemplate and meditate, not on the current state of worldly affairs, but of our own internal landscape?

Our lives have been brilliantly compartmentalized— honeycombed to death with routine, expectations, laws, regulations, and the insatiable desire to succeed at the expense of our wellbeing. Society has run amok! And we're stuck in the mud and mire of a system that breeds fearful men to fill the slots, like horses to be released from stalls and race to their last breath. Can we not see the monopoly game we're trapped in? Do you not feel the strings dictating your every move, constantly pulling and pushing you to serve a predetermined agenda?

The true enemy is not from any external force, but from within. We, believing that our small, limited, weak selves must work hard to ingratiate deeper into a system that will eventually reward us with money, fame, and fine objects if we can just work hard and long enough – *obediently enough* – without making too much trouble – without asking too many questions – simply shutting up and getting busy, and taking the paycheck to buy food and get drunk on weekends to have sufficiently destroyed enough braincells to do it all over again—for another week; another year; another decade;

and for most of us, another lifetime.

Samsara, the continuous wheel of death and rebirth, destined to spin over and over and over, lest one wakes up— not only in their waking lives, but also in their dreaming ones. You mustn't be content to sleep another thousand years. It's your choice of free will, but a job that you'll have to tackle sooner or later. It may feel good to sleep, but to be awake is to be alive. Allow mate to be your *dream yoga,* as you practice daily to remain awake and aware. Know thyself.

> *Drinking tea is most valued when there are few guests; where there is a multitude of people there is clamor; when there is clamor tasteful interest is lacking! Solitary sipping is called peaceful; two guests are called elegant; three to four people are called a delight; five to six people are called common; seven to eight people are called depraved.*[2]
> - RECORD OF TEA, ZHANG YUAN

Drinking mate alone is just as good as drinking it with others. While with friends you'll form an external circle; while alone, the circle will form within. Break your daily routine with your mate and sit for awhile to reflect on your internal climate and refract the stress, drama, and bullshit you experience daily.

Learn from the soothing, pulsating wave that rides through your nervous system as the mate enters your biology and tethers to your nerves with tentacles of wisdom and peace and clarity. The herb is doing its best to show you Her face; but you, too, must try and *see* Her.

Let go of your worries and accept things as they are, allowing the storm to settle and equilibrium to reinstate itself in your spirit. Remain still and the muses will come and form a circle around you. The lone wolf is never alone. Plug into the Source and draw energy from each sip. Your bombilla is not a straw, but a bridge to a pool of wisdom far beyond the perimeter of your gourd.

Fill your gourd and see where the water meets the brim. This is the ocean; the infinitely deep well that drops through the gourd, through the Earth, extinguishing the Hells of your inner demons, and coming full circle through your next breath. Exhale the rainbow. When you watch with a child's eye as your water comes to a small boil, do not see the steam of the kettle, but see the God of Water taking the misty, ethereal form, preparing to once again embrace the herb she last saw in the fields, by the farmer's hand. Now pour your thermos and flow the fountain of youth. Not a step of mate shall be taken as ordinary. Each sip; each slurp; each pour; each gaze into the gourd; each whiff; each adjustment of the bombilla; each thought that arises is holy. You are *not* insignificant!

You may think that you chose to drink mate, but I say: mate has equally chosen you. I can't tell you how many times I had offered someone mate and observed them sheepishly sip the bombilla as if I dipped it in the Ebola virus: with one eye on the gourd and the other on me, as if to say "you better not be poisoning me, man!" We're like flowers, only open to the new when the full light of sun exposes every detail, and closed at the first sight of darkness—the first inkling of stepping into the unknown. Could we be any more fickle? We're too fast to turn away from the Light. Some men have healed themselves from disease solely by staring into the sun. "Sun Gazing"[3] is what they're calling it. Just ask HRM.

Mate in North American Culture

Powerful compounds called saponins account for mate's bitterness. When the mate is no longer bitter, it has become washed, *lavado*. The bitterness is a reliable indicator of the mate's potency to heal: when there's no longer taste, you've depleted the healing energy of the herb, and it's time to change the mate.

The first few times I had mate, the bitterness of it quickly led me to add sugar, honey, and agave. Those were my training wheels. If it's meant to be, you and mate will form a bond and forever be inextricably united. But there's a dance at first. Being so accustomed to our coffee, tea, and soda, we've stiffened our necks to stare straight ahead. The prescriptions of the society. Drink this. Eat that. Healthy this. Unhealthy that. Yet all the while it's only a few who benefit from these arbitrary lines.

Then comes the issue of the North American temperament towards *sharing* mate. Most Americans (excuse me if I omit the "North" for brevity) shun at the thought of sharing a straw with their own brothers, let alone *several times with a complete stranger.*

To be fair, however, there are some who wouldn't think twice to share a *bombilla,* the straw with a filter used for drinking mate. I speak generally here. The average American, seeing the bombilla jammed into one mouth after another, immediately thinks of "getting a cold" or "catching a stomach virus."

I used to think the same. But after three-years of sharing innumerable bombillas, I can attest to you that I'm well and healthy—hardly ever getting sick. Besides, spreading germs from mouth to mouth has a way of building the immune system, not hampering it. I can't imagine most people thinking about catching a cold before they kiss someone.

Americans, as a whole, lack a cultural drink. Not out of intention, but a result of our wide and deep diversity of cultures and backgrounds. We have our joints, beer, and wine as the rest of the countries, but not a drink that we could really call our own.

I'm not proposing mate or any other drink to fill such a void, nor would I be opposed to the idea. If it happened naturally, so be it. I believe in ten-years, mate will have pervaded every facet of our American society. There will be mate lounges; medicine; supplements; pills; foods; weight loss drinks; smoothies; shakes; injections? you name it. Perhaps this very book will be a catalyst for such proliferation.

Mate will be a part of the Coming of Age of our relatively young nation. I'm not speaking of technology or advances in industry – we're already on the forefront of those – but of the gross lack of spiritual expression.

What we have in money and military, we lack in spirituality and a profound sense of community. Yes, there are pockets here and there – towns that show you nothing but love and openness – but pants only have four pockets.

Mate will help us build such values and compassion between one another. To sit, as equals, for a moment, forgetting that he is "black" or she is "white" or they are

42

"yellow", and simply coming together for a few mates under one roof. We have a lot to learn from South America in this regard. To take your time – forgetting about the rush for a few minutes – and partake in something that goes beyond class, race, socioeconomic status.

My job is to continue spreading the *symbol* of mate. About the it's-more-than-a-drink aspect that is not always easily seen with a critical, fixed eye. Gaze at mate, don't stare. See the auroral intelligence that escapes each gourd and penetrates each mote. Let its influence draw you nearer and nearer, until she's got you close. Who could have known that such a drink ever existed.

Sometimes it's a matter of nudging someone towards their first gourd. Grassy herb floating in some sort of plant container, doesn't always scream "sexy!" But once the herb is allowed to play in the body, mind, and spirit, that's when the real magic begins. How many times have I heard people say "at first I didn't like it, but now I drink it daily; weird." Not weird—magic.

When I first came to Argentina in '09, I recall a girlfriend of mine. Her parents would always offer me healthy servings of olive oil, madly drenching my dishes—salads, rices, pizza, you name it. At first, not being accustomed to so much olive oil, and certainly not olives, I had some resistance. But they persisted, and I allowed them to serve me the best way they knew how.

Upon returning to New York for several months, the first day home, I remember having an unusual craving for black olives. Scouring the fridge, I found a bottle and ate them all. Delicious, smooth, round, creamy. I inhaled them. The following days I found myself copiously glazing my dishes with olive oil. I thought: "it was only a few short months ago that I couldn't stand the taste of olives and seldom used it apart from frying, never in its crude form." And there I was, absolutely loving everything that olives had to offer. A superfood, indeed.

The body has a way of knowing what it needs, even if your ego doesn't. I believe that same holistic metamorphosis occurs with mate: at first you may resist, but in time it'll catch up to you. And later, it'll be *you* who's doing the chasing!

Perhaps we should call mate the Kitchen Drink, *Mate Cocina*. How many times have I shared mates, intimately, with a good friend in my kitchen. There's a magic about the kitchen. Something to do with the small spaces here in Argentina, where the kitchens are no more than several feet across by several feet wide. A mate nest.

Mate made in the kitchen seems wanting to remain

there. It feels comfortable standing near the kettle and stove. I like when people take a seat on the countertops and pass the gourd above the shallow kitchen tiles. Mate flourishes in the waves between our heart-to-heart transmission; who is speaking to whom is of no consequence. The mate revels in this revere. It's her world. It's where she was conceived. At that moment, we cease to put mate in ourselves, but step inside of mate, ourselves. Mate will cook our hearts open. Conversations stir like batter. The yerba leavens our minds.

You'll find your own favorite spot to drink mate. Some love to drink outside in parks; in their living rooms; at work; alone in the morning. The mate will be drunk where it resides. Whether that be at work, while doing your accounting, or at home, while writing your poetry—alone on the patio. Some will shun the lone mate drinker, casting him off as antisocial or unfriendly. But I assure you, that that's the furthest from the case.

Drinking mate alone has been one of my greatest rituals. If I drink alone, I practice infinity of Self. If I drink within a circle, I join my inner 0 with theirs and form ∞. Let there be no calculation of the holy holly herb! Let no question of race or money or fame sour our yerba.

Water is the most impressionable substance on Earth, the medium in which the essence of the yerba is expressed;

however, it's the *purity of heart* – responsible for the *true* taste and experience of mate, coaxing the herb to its maximum potential – that completes the Circle.

There are no hard rules with mate. We keep the traditions as well as create our own, simultaneously. A flexible drink. You host your mate circle however, and with whomever you resonate with. Maybe you'll share mate while you philosophize on life. Or maybe you'll serve it with *medialunas de manteca,* glazed croissants, to sweeten the circle. Maybe you'll add sugar or agave or honey; or keep it simple and *amargo.* Maybe you'll sit in your room or in your kitchen. Remember, the real state of mate has nothing to do with the real estate where it's drunk.

I drink more mate alone than I do with friends. And the journey continues. Everything that mate is, now becomes everything that I am. It's a marriage; a symbiosis. A gathering of old friends for another round of building and progressing. This is the genius of mate that lies beyond the microscope and prodding instruments of the scientist. It's of no part, but the whole. The closer we look, the further away it'll get from understanding. To participate in a mate circle and allow mate to do what it does, is enough.

Just yesterday, I hosted several circles in my apartment.

A friend of mine, a translator, begun reading a book about mate called *El Mate, Bebida Nacional Argentina,* by Francisco N. Scutellá.

As she translated from castellano to English, I sat, mesmerized and enchanted, in my own world, listening to wonderful mate-infused prose.

Where am I? What place have I been transported to. Who are these people that I sit with and laugh and converse and love with? What is this circle that has formed? How did this come about?

Cool wind blowing from the gaping windows. I can smell the ash from the spent cigars and cigarettes. Smiles. Lounging around. Listening. Interacting. Equally communing with words and silence. I can't help but feel unequivocally happy.

What problems do I have? Where are my worries? To whom can I blame for anything? Right, I'm deeply steeped in the mate. I'm infused with magic and invigorated with the same strength that allows the dandelion to explode through the asphalt. I can imagine no more complete circle in the world. Take a seat, Giotto.

The Server Remains Low

As the server, never lose your purity of heart. Your vibrations must be of such a high frequency, that you pick everyone up off their feet. Which is also to say, you remain the lowest, most meek, humble servant.

Only in service to others can you rise as the steam does each gourd. Only in accordance to the one and only law, Love, can you truly participate in the circle. There's an anonymous saying *"No se puede tomar mate si se está enojado,"* you can't drink mate when you're mad. And how true this is! For mate is the rainbow on your gray sky. Let it shine, let it shine, let it shine!

Allow Grace to penetrate every cubic inch of your body, and every etheric inch of your spirit. I can now see, with my mind's eye, why mate was called "The Drink of the Gods," because every sip invites you to sit around a God. Every circle gives you the chance to *be* God.

It has never been more necessary than now, to recognize the importance of coming together and sharing—sharing whatever it may be. In our case, mate. But you can now see that mate is nothing more than the symbol, the placeholder. The grand metaphor of Unity.

Chapter 4

Mateware

Getting Started

Everything that's used to prepare and enjoy mate is your mateware:

1. Gourd, frenchpress, or teapot.
2. Loose-leaf yerba (herb).
3. Bombilla.
4. Thermos.
5. Kettle.

A Look at Mate Terminology

Let's begin by setting the mate jargon straight. "Mate" (pronounced MAH-tay) is the term traditionally used to describe the entire unit: bombilla, gourd, and yerba.

So when we say, "let's drink some mate," we are saying, "set everything up: heat the water, add the yerba, and place the bombilla... *Vamos!*" What is produced is the "mate."

"Want to drink a few mates?" is a common question here in Argentina. The plural, "mates", now being used to describe what I call a "cycle", or simply, a round of mate. The cycle is a "turn" that someone takes to drink the mate, then ending that turn with an audible – and *quite acceptable – ssslllluuuurrrrpppppp!!!!* Signifying that you are satisfied and have finished the entire gourd, down to the last sip.

"Yerba" (pronounced: yer-BAH) is the castellano word for herb. So technically, there are all sorts of yerbas: mint, tea, basil, fennel, etc. Yerba, in our case, is the actual mate leaves, stems, and dust that we add to our gourd.

The gourd is the mate cup. But here's where it gets a bit confusing. "Mate" is *also* the name for just the "gourd" or "cup". So if you ask someone on the streets (of Argentina) "where can I get a mate?" they'll, correctly, think you're asking "where can I purchase a gourd" not *yerba*.

It doesn't go beyond that. Outside of South America, "mate" is usually considered just the herb. In the States when we say "let's drink mate, man!" we're saying, let's make a gourd and drink mate. And if you say, "where can I get some mate?" we're referring to the herb, not what the Argentines would consider the gourd (mate).

Selecting Your Mateware

The Gourd (Mate)

The first thing you want to do is get yourself a good gourd. There are two principal fashions: wooden and calabash. The latter is made from the hollowed and dried-out end of the *calabash* (squash). When fully dried, a metal brim is sometimes added, allowing the bombilla to sit nicely.

Wooden gourds are usually made with two sorts of wood: *palo santo*, holy stick, and *algarrobo*, carob. I'm partial to wooden gourds, because they're easier to maintain and keep dry. The slightly scented sappy wood tends to gently increase the aromatics of the yerba. Gourds made from palo santo give off a piney scent that enhances the flavor of the yerba.

Carob gourds, made with soft reddish wood, impart a mild oaky flavor. The carob wood is also significantly less dense, resulting in a lighter gourd. But what you gain in lightness, you lose in heat protection, as this gourd allows the heat to more easily pass through the wood and potentially burn or heat-up your hand if the water temperature is too high. Nevertheless, the carob gourd has been a mainstay within my circles, and I have found that most people like them. Spanish cedar is also an acceptable wood for gourds.

Fashion is on the rise within the mate community as we are seeing more and more *chic* gourds hitting the market: glass, metal, silicone, ceramic, etc.

Experiment with the gourd that's right for you. In any case, if you go with a plant-based gourd (wooden or squash), you'll have to properly cure it before use; we'll discuss that in a second, but first let me explain, in more detail, some of the pros and cons of each.

Wooden

These gourds are versatile and easy to prepare mate. They usually have a nice scent, imparted from the tree's lingering resins. They're often perfectly shaped for good gripping, with a nicely curved brim that allows you to neatly wrap your fingers for optimal handling.

The cons with wooden gourds are that they are smaller, so hold less yerba. Some prefer to use the larger, more traditional calabash gourds when hosting a circle. From my experience, though, using larger gourds, especially the gigantic ones typical of Brazil, can often be intimidating to new mate drinkers. I can't tell you how many times I've heard *"do I have to finish this whole thing?"*

However, if you were to visit Uruguay, it would be sacrilegious not to be using a large calabash or ceramic gourd, which is typically used in that region.

Having spent several years in Buenos Aires, I have become accustomed to the smaller wooden gourds, or the *Palermo gourds*, that I affectionately call them. Palermo is a fashionable district in the heart of the city; you'll see many people there drinking from small gourds.

Some wooden varieties are prone to cracking—closely monitor the curing process for forming splits in the wood.

Calabash

Nothing is more traditional than the calabash gourd. From times of antiquity, indigenous peoples have been using the calabash as a vessel for yerba; it's inextricably tied to the tradition and meaning of mate, and I expect it'll remain so.

In United States, as of 2012, we are starting to see a rise in these gourds—they are more available than their wooden counterparts.

These gourds come in various sizes and shapes and can easily be purchased from online mate retailers as well as street vendors in Argentina, Uruguay, and Brazil.

The main issue I have with these gourds is the unavoidable

excess of plant matter that lingers at the base. You'll notice a peeling effect of the calabash rind upon curing, sometimes lasting up to several weeks. It's advised to scrape out as much as this plant skin as possible, so as not to affect the taste of the yerba, or worse, be drawn through the bombilla.

In time you'll *usually* be able to get rid of all the skin— and smoothen the natural honeycomb-like texture with constant use. Allow your gourd to fully dry after each use, preventing mold. If mold forms, which is usual and nothing to worry about, completely dry out the gourd for 2–3 days, while it rests on its side.

As with tobacco pipes, you'll want to have at least two gourds at your disposal, constantly alternating between a drying gourd and one in use—especially for someone hosting several mate ceremonies per week.

Ceramic

I recently purchased a ceramic gourd in Colonia, Uruguay. Not surprisingly, I bought it from an aisle devoted solely to mate in a supermarket. *Can you imagine?*

In Argentina and Uruguay, there are literally shelves towering with yerba; coffee occupies a small portion of the space—the exact opposite of the United States, where coffee is dominant.

The gourd was beautifully encased in red leather. Heavy, but just right. Warm to the touch. Comfy. I use this ceramic gourd at least once, every time I get a new yerba—allowing me to taste the *true* essence of the mate, without any imparting flavors from the wooden or calabash gourds.

If you appreciate mate like a fine wine or gourmet coffee, as I do, then have at least one glass or ceramic gourd.

The aesthetics of the ceramic gourd gives off a certain regal display. It's a nice change-up if you only have a wooden or calabash gourd. Though, I must admit that no matter how many new gourds I accumulate, I always go back to my simple wooden mate. What can I say, I'm a simple man.

The main issue you'll find with ceramics is the silicone underlining of the brim that's meant to act as a seal between the attached metal top and the ceramic. I find that the yerba sometimes gets stuck there in the fine line, even when the gourd is totally washed-out. In order to remove the yerba, you have to fill it with water and place your hand above the top of the gourd and give it a few hard shakes.

Silicone

Silicone gourds are one of the latest entries to the circle. Molded from food-grade silicone, they are impervious to heat and won't melt when hot water is added.

They are good for quick use and are very easy to clean when changing yerba—nothing sticks inside. An ideal mate for someone not greatly interested in having to cure their gourd and keep it dry.

Offices and shops that have mate-drinking employees will soon catch-on to these new, easy-to-use gourds. With a few rinses, they are completely washed and ready to dry or be used again. I foresee a lot of young, new Materos using them. Who knows, drinking mate may even become *fashionable*.

How to Cure Your Gourd

Below, I will describe the most generally accepted and recognized method—the one that I learned from Argentines. Both wooden and calabash gourds apply, but take note that you may want to scrape out the inside flakes of the calabash gourd after it's fully cured.

1. Rinse out your new gourd with fresh cold water.

2. Fill your gourd ¾ with yerba mate.
3. Add properly heated mate water (160–180°F) to your gourd—fill to the brim.
4. Let the gourd sit for 24 hours, occasionally topping it off with room temperature water every several hours.

Curing the gourd ensures that it'll last as long as it possibly can—perhaps for several years if properly cared for. Visible and microscopic holes and cracks are sealed in this process, as the gourd absorbs the water and expands, tightening the organic material, preventing cracking and leaking over time.

I've heard of people curing their gourds with whisky. You could cure your gourd with just about any liquid that you enjoy: vodka, brandy, wine, bourbon, etc. Though, be careful not to cure it with a flavor that you'll regret smelling or tasting. It'll take some time for the curing liquid, if it's other than water, to completely leave your gourd. I recommend pure water.

The Bombilla

Pronounced "bom-BEE-yah," the word literally means "straw" in castellano. Without the bombilla, there's no drinking mate. It's an essential tool when drinking mate the traditional way. Unless you're drinking *mate cocido*, tea bags, or mate in a frenchpress, then drinking mate will be impossible without your trusted bombilla.

With bombilla styles you have a few options: fanned, coiled, spoon, chambered, double-action, pick, and bamboo or wooden. Most bombillas nowadays have some degree of curvature, as to prevent the Matero from having to lower their head unnecessarily and uncomfortably while drinking.

In the book *El Mate,* by Argentine Mate Extraordinaire, Scutellá, we learn of the Italian immigrant, Annio Silvio Pizzoni, having come to live in Buenos Aires after WWI to work as a taxi driver.

One day, observing the straight line of the bombillas in use, he decided to make a curved bombilla which became a conversation piece with his clients. Later, he would begin manufacturing them and so began the invention—or at least one invention story, of the prevalent curved bombillas we see today.[1]

Fanned Bombilla

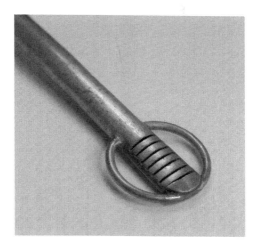

The fanned bombilla has a ring around the end of the filter, with small horizontal slits. They have more resistance, which I prefer. It helps me to better appreciate the taste, as less liquid enters my mouth. It's like smoking a perfect cigar with the right amount of tension: if it permits too much smoke, it's overwhelming; too little, it's difficult.

One of the best things about the fanned bombilla is that you can better maneuver the yerba in the gourd when it needs to be repositioned—if it becomes *tapado,* clogged, or you need to fix the angle.

It's also better for scraping out the yerba when you're on to your next round of mates: the fan-like shape of the bombilla acts like a shovel's head allowing you to scoop. You can't quite achieve that with the cylindrical, coiled bombilla.

Coiled Bombilla

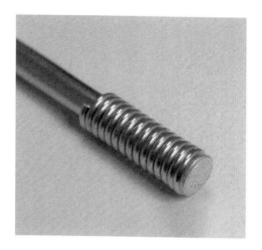

We never forget our *first*. For me, it was the standard coiled bombilla. As a coil tightly rung together acting as a filter, it's the most simple modern bombilla. The liquid enters through the fine slivers between the coils and the yerba is kept out.

These bombillas are usually stainless steel, not made of the superior alpaca metal. Problematic at times is the cap that's on the bottom of the coil: it's usually made from generic metal and tends to corrode. Look for one that's completely stainless.

61

Spoon Bombilla

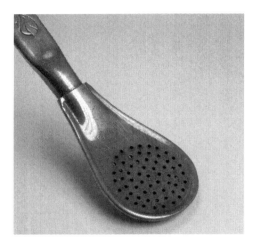

The spoon bombilla is my favorite. For someone that drinks plenty of finely cut Gaucho mate, it's indispensable. With a spoon-shaped filter dotted with pin-sized holes, it's the perfect bombilla to scoop under the thicker, more spongy Gaucho yerbas that tend to cake-up inside the gourd.

These bombillas are common in Uruguay and Brazil. Sometimes the spoon bombilla's shaft is flattened instead of retaining a roundness like other bombillas. Some prefer flat bombillas because they are easier to sip and naturally sit on the lips.

Double Action Bombilla™ *(Spring Loaded)*

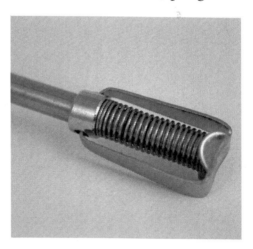

This is an interesting double-take on the coiled and spoon bombilla. The bombilla has several holes at the end, which are covered with a spring that acts as a second filtered layer; that spring is affixed to the end of the bombilla with an adjustable wing-like wrapper that pins the isolated spring over the holes beneath.

This bombilla is more typical of Argentina, though, in Uruguay, you're likely to see a different version of this bombilla where the entire filter mechanism is fused together as opposed to moveable parts.

Chambered Bombilla

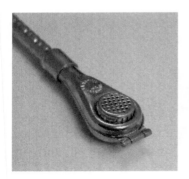 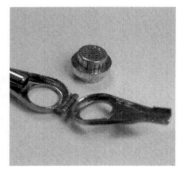

This awkward bombilla has a tea-ball-like chamber encased inside a latch that swings open like a door. The chamber is placed inside the enclosure then the door is swung back down, and the entire filter is locked into place with a small metal ring that wraps around the enclosure's handle, firmly securing the filter to the bombilla.

Apart from the cumbersome nature of this bombilla, the chamber tends to rattle as you sip the yerba, which makes for an annoying vibration. Some Materos love this bombilla; some hate it. The movable parts are too many; simplicity is sacrificed for an overly-mechanized and clumsy design which may *look* cool, but doesn't quite work so well.

Pick Bombilla

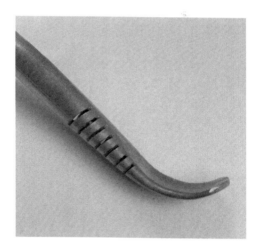

I call this bombilla a pick because it's shaped like the dental picks used during a cleaning. Usually made from alpaca, it has an acute bend, or "pick," as the filter, with several fine slivers across each side. The pick is especially good for scraping out the flesh of the calabash gourd during the curing process. It's also very handy for simply spooning-out used yerba.

Bamboo Bombilla

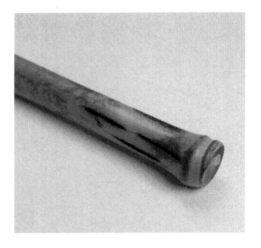

Made from a thin and slightly bent bamboo cane, this bombilla is most in accord with Nature. Though not as common as the metal ones, these bombillas are appealing. You may also find wooden bombillas, but are equally out-of-fashion with the modern Matero. If you grow bamboo, try making your own by cutting a thin portion of a cane and boring pinholes into the base for a natural filter.

Mate Thermos

A mate thermos keeps your water at the right temperature. If you're serious about mate, you'll need one. Remember: the water *makes* the mate.

If it's too cool, the mate will never open and bloom to its full potential of flavors. If too hot, it'll kill the mate before you get a chance to experience it—mate abhors boiling water. If the water has chlorine, then your mate is dead before the first sip.

Mate enjoys hot water, but not hot enough to boil. Once you achieve such a temperature, 160–180°F, you'll need a good stainless steel thermos to maintain the heat.

A quality thermos will hold the heat for several hours before the water gets cold. Any local Kmart, Ikea, or Target will have dependable thermoses for under $20. Don't be afraid to get yourself two if you plan to drink mate in the park with friends—ensuring that you have enough water for a few hours of circles. It's best to get the standard 1L thermos, nothing smaller.

You can also purchase an airpot, traditionally used to serve coffee at delis and cafes to store up to 1 gallon of mate water for those long circles lasting several hours.

Mate Kettle

Get yourself a hardy stainless steel, 1L kettle. Kettles come in different shapes and sizes. Choose one that fits your style.

Since a large part of preparing mate is the experience of carefully watching the water, and making sure that it doesn't reach a boil, I prefer kettles with large top openings. When the water is getting close to its perfect temperature, I remove the top and keep a close eye on what's going on inside, making sure to remove the kettle at the right time.

If you host mate circles, then you may consider getting a larger kettle, of at least 2L capacity so you can fill two thermoses.

You'll also find electric kettles that allow you to set the temperature. I've experimented with these, but I find that they aren't too precise in achieving the right temperature. No machine can replace the human senses. Besides, I rather like standing around the kettle and immersing myself fully in the joy of preparing mate. In a way, I become another tool, as I determine *just the right* temperature. However, if you're pressed for time and just want to get down to *business,* then going electric is suitable.

Caring for your Mateware

Don't share when you're sick

Is there need to worry about getting sick from sharing your mate? A reasonable question. If you're sick, it's best not to share mate, nor accept the invitation to join a circle. Common courtesy prevails here—use your own best judgement.

Keep Your Gourd Dry

Keep your mateware as dry and clean as possible when not in use. The gourd should fully dry before the next use, allowing it to naturally disinfect. Occasionally, for additional disinfection, allow fully boiled water to remain in the gourd for several minutes.

Boiling your bombillas

As for keeping the bombilla clean, wash it like you would any plate, with mild detergent and soft sponge; this helps keep the alpaca and stainless steel lustrous and shiny.

It's a good idea to boil all of your bombillas once a week for at least 10 minutes, fully eliminating any risk of bacteria and *curing the bombilla* by removing inner debris.

Kettle Care

If you wash your kettle with soap, make sure it's a mild detergent. Preferably, if the kettle begins to accumulate minerals or residue, wash it by boiling a bit of salt and lemon juice, then scour it out. Optionally, scrub the inside with baking soda then rinse well.

Storing Your Mateware

Gourd

Keep your mateware in a cool and well-aerated location. Some people like to hang their gourds upside-down, or tilt them on a downward angle for all the water to drain. That's optional, but not necessary; just make sure never to let a pool of water sit in your gourd—that'd be a perfect breeding ground for bacteria. By having two gourds to alternate between, you'll always have a dry one available.

Yerba

You can keep the yerba in the original bag and simply roll the top over or use a large paperclip (used to bind screenplays) to secure it. It can be stored in any of the following: baking tins, sealable plastic bags, and a glass jar.

If you store in glass, keep out of direct sunlight. Keep the mate in a cool, dry, dark location—just as you would store loose-leaf tea or ground coffee beans.

Your Mateware is Sacred

You have your gourd, your bombilla, your kettle, your thermos, and, *of course,* your favorite yerba! This is your mateware. When you have all these essentials, you're set.

Store everything in a dry, cool location, as we've discussed. Keep everything as clean as you can—periodically sterilizing your bombillas by boiling them for a few minutes. Find some good tins for your yerba and don't be shy about getting a few gourds—experiment between calabash, wood, metal, and ceramic. Have at least two bombillas— as mentioned earlier, you have coiled, fanned, and spoon bombillas. Try all. I carry a few bombillas to circles because the bombilla gets "stale" after several cycles, when the tip becomes sticky and bits of yerba may start clinging to it. When this happens, I usually don't try to clean it and, instead, opt to replace it entirely.

Your mateware is sacred—tools, helping to bring people together; keep them in impeccable order. When you're done drinking for the day, empty your mate (for the compost or plant fertilizer) and let your gourd dry for the night; it'll be ready and fresh for the next day of mates.

Chapter 5

Preparing and Serving Mate

The person serving mate shouldn't be the one who has the desire,
but the one who knows how to serve.
- FRANCISCO SCUTELLÁ

Water was boiled in a cauldron while the correct temperature of the
boil was determined by viewing the bubbles forming in the pot.
Just at the right moment, milled tea powder was added...[1]
- THE ANCIENT ART OF TEA

Preparing mate is equally art as ritual. It's the opening of the mate experience, where people gather around the kettle as one prepares the water and others, usually slyly lurking close by, warning "don't boil the water."

In Argentina, nearly every time I'm preparing water for a circle, one person gives me this friendly warning to make sure to watch the water. *"Cuidado, eh...?"* It's something said more out of friendly habit than genuine advice.

And the dance continues as I pour a bit of cold water *(dummy water)* into the gourd to prevent the mate from being burned, then patiently waiting to see the small bubbles forming at the base of the kettle and the water swirling with heatwaves as the perfect temperature of around 175°F is reached—then on to adding the hot water into the waterhole opposing the mountain of mate that was formed on one side of the gourd while inverting and shaking it against my palm, then finally placing the bombilla on the opposite side of the gourd, straight down across from the opposing downward angle of the yerba, creating a rough 45° angle; then onto drinking the first one or two mates (dummy mates), as the server, to ensure the fine quality and temperature before passing in on to my guests, or continuing to drink if I'm alone.

Mate Water

The inherent quality of tea must be expressed in water. When a tea that is an eight meets with water that is a ten, the tea is also a ten! When water that is an eight pairs with a tea that is a ten then the tea is just an eight.[2]

- THE ANCIENT ART OF TEA

Excellent mate has as much, *if not more,* to do with the quality of water as the quality of yerba. The water is the current in which the mate's flavor and characteristics and healing properties are expressed—it is the vehicle the mate travels through.

The water you use to prepare your mate must be pure and free from chemicals such as chlorine, that damage the water's ability to remain intact and pristine. If your water isn't pure, such as unfiltered or poor quality bottled water, your mate experience can only go so far.

If you were seeking a diamond, would you settle for a pile of hardened dirt?

If you want to truly experience the power of mate, don't settle for poor water quality just because you're used to using tap water. The chemicals in the tap have already diminished the water's life force.

Dr. Masaru Emoto, known for his groundbreaking work on exploring how crystals form in water – determined by either positive or negative vibrations – teaches us that water from poor sources are always compromised and not in alignment with Nature:

We can surmise that when a complete geometric crystal is formed, water is in alignment with nature and the phenomenon we call life. The crystals do not form in water that has been polluted by the results of our failure to remember the laws of nature. When we tried taking photographs of crystals from Tokyo's tap water, the results were pitiful. This is because the water is sanitized with chlorine, thus damaging the innate ability of the water to form crystals.[3]

The study of ancient tea masters reveal how much time, patience, and art was put into locating and selecting the finest water.

You needn't go on an excursion to find naturally erupting spring water in the woods, though with findaspring.com, it's entirely possible. However, by purchasing a few gallons of spring water or investing in a high quality water filter that's been proven, without a doubt, to be effective, you will ensure that your mate remains on a high caliber, resulting in the best possible experience for you and your Materos.

Heating Mate Water

Carefully watching the water like a hawk, ready to steal the kettle from its flame at the first sight of the smallest bubbles popping forth, I remain vigilant in the art of preparing mate water.

The Ancient Chinese Tea Master, Lu Yu, attests to "Three Boils," varying in intensity of heat and size of bubbles:

Of boiling, when the boiling water is like fish eyes, and there is a slight noise, this is the first boil. When on the edges it is like a surging spring and joined pearls, this is the second boil. When the water is surging and swelling waves (rolling boil), this is the third boil. Anything after this, the water is old and cannot be drunk.[4]

You'll want to get your water somewhere between the first and second boils. The first boil will appear to be like large grains of sand, or "crab eyes"[4] as the Chinese describe. The second boil shows slightly larger bubbles, like small pebbles. Once you see the "crab eyes" appear, wait several seconds just as they begin to slightly increase in size, then remove the kettle and pour your mate water into your thermos. If you outright boil the water, then it's old and dead—useless for mate.

Adding Yerba to Your Gourd

With the highest grade yerba at your disposal, it's time to fill your gourd.

1. Fill your gourd between ½ to ¾ full of yerba. Experiment

with the amount. Gaucho cuts usually do better with a ½ full gourd, since the powdery yerba expands. The less viscous Argentine cuts prefer ¾ capacity.

2. Take your gourd with one hand and completely cover the top with the palm of your opposing hand; invert the gourd on a downward angle and shake it in a downward-upward motion. While returning the gourd to normal position, create a 45° angle on the yerba—this is called your *mountain of mate.* Opposing your mountain of mate, you should now have a cavity to place your water; this is called your *waterhole.*

Why shake the yerba? This process not only creates the necessary waterhole for you to place your bombilla and add your water, but also brings the small dust particles to the top and keeps the larger stems and leaves below, acting as a natural filter and preventing your bombilla from becoming clogged.

Some new drinkers shake the mate to futilely remove all of the dust—mistakenly thinking that it's not to be drunk. But the dust is an essential ingredient to any good mate, and it's not to be removed, apart from the small amount that's retained on your palm.

Now set your gourd aside and gather your dummy water.

Dummy Water for Dummy Mates

The term "dummy" is not stated offensively, but rather signifying an honor to drink the first two, underprepared, mates for the sake of the circle.

After the dummy water – cold or, preferably, room-temperature – has been added, the server drinks the first dummy mate, then he adds a second dummy water for the second dummy mate that he drinks as well, ensuring the quality of the mates to be served, considering: heat, taste, bombilla placement, etc.

Dummy water is added to protect the vital nutrients of the yerba as well as preventing the delicate herb from being scorched by the fully heated water. Effectively, the dummy water tempers the yerba. Below you'll see how to prepare the dummy mates:

1. Carefully maintaining your mountain of mate, start adding your dummy water to your gourd's waterhole. Let this water absorb into the yerba for 1 minute.
2. After your yerba has absorbed the dummy water, place your bombilla and drink your first official dummy mate.
3. Now add more dummy water and drink your second dummy mate.

Positioning the Bombilla

Place your bombilla across from the downward angle of yerba; the spout should have its back to the mountain of yerba; it should slip right in, but if you have to, don't be afraid to adjust it in the perfect position that suits you. We often hear "don't touch the bombilla!" But, as the server, you may touch the bombilla and adjust as needed.

Depending on the style of bombilla, there are particular ways to position them in the gourd.

Over the mountain

Fanned and coiled bombillas should be laid over the yerba instead of scooping under the yerba. The slits should be facing the wall of the gourd, never the yerba. You will be "drinking over the mountain" of yerba in this case.

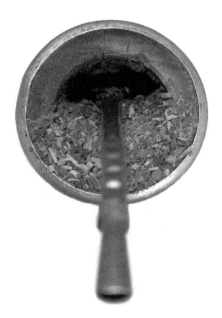

Under the mountain

If you're using a spoon bombilla, then scoop it under the yerba; you will not be drinking over, but "under the mountain." This is usually the case with pick, spoon, and double action bombillas. However, the only bombillas that are scooped under the yerba are ones with a curved filter: pick and spoon; it would be near impossible to do it with any other.

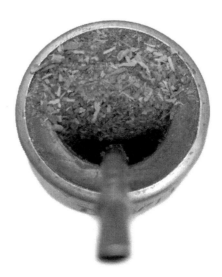

Testing the Mate's Quality

Time to test the mate. Being from the States you may think it rude not to prepare the mate then immediately pass it to your guests – as one would do in any normal social setting – but with mate, being "rude" is actually being "polite."

As the server of the mate, it's your duty, solemnly sworn to the Gods of Mate, with your right hand raised to the Holy Gourd, to drink the first one or two mates and promise to forever ensure the most perfect, pristine, superb mate, lest you die and awake in yerba purgatory.

If the water is too cold, back to the kettle and heat another pot. If the water is too hot and scolding – you guessed it – back to the kettle for a new batch of water. Attaining that sweet spot between 160 and 180°F will become an art in and of itself.

As straightforward as preparing a good mate may *appear,* there are many seemingly little, but tremendously vital, things that can go wrong. Once you find your rhythm, through continued practice, you'll know what to do like it's second nature. But still, you'll have to remain sharp and steady—constantly honing the skills of a Matero.

Mate Serving Etiquette

Generally, Only the Server is to Adjust the Bombilla

When the quality of the mate has been thoroughly vetted – *then, and only then* – refill the gourd and pass it to the person to your right.

Brace yourself, for what you may see next can produce feelings of rage, shock, and the sudden urge to pull your eyes out of their sockets: the neophyte drinker may begin to stir the bombilla as one would stir a cube of sugar in tea. A perfect opportunity to explain yerba mate serving and drinking traditions.

Passing the Mate

This is your ceremony, so treat it as such. Tell your guests that when they're done with the mate, pass it back to *you*, the server, so that you can prepare another mate and pass it on to the next person.

The server is always the hinge to the door: everything opens and closes with her. She prepares the mate; tests the mate; passes it to the guests; receives the finished mate; makes another mate; then passes it on to the next; and when the yerba becomes tasteless or the thermos runs dry, it's, again, the server's happy duty to prepare more water and add new yerba to the gourd.

The server is running the show, but no more or less important than any Matero in the circle.

Changing Lavado Yerba

When the yerba becomes tasteless, it's considered washed *(lavado)*. It's now time to dump the yerba and prepare a new mate.

The best indicators of determining when your mate is washed, besides it becoming tasteless, is when you no longer see white, foamy bubbles on the surface, and the yerba appears to be waterlogged—at this stage, all the "good stuff" has been depleted and your mate is spent.

Mate Serving Tricks

Waterhole

This is the hole where you add your mate water to the gourd. It's good to maintain some space around your bombilla; it shouldn't be too cemented into the yerba, which will diminish your ability, as the server, to flex and adjust the bombilla to ensure that it doesn't become clogged, or *tapado.*

Keep your waterhole clean. As the yerba becomes *lavado,* your waterhole will eventually become a new mountain of mate as you switch the hemispheres of your bombilla (more on that soon).

Mate Molding

When drinking Gaucho and Paraguayan cuts, mate molding comes in handy. Using a spoon bombilla, you can mold your mountain of mate and secure it firmly against the wall of the gourd. This allows for you to keep your waterhole clear and prevents clogging. And most importantly, it keeps your mountain of mate intact for when you need it later.

Bombilla Hemisphere Switching

The bombilla always begins in Argentina, the southern hemisphere. This isn't meant to be taken literally, as either side of the mate is fine to place your bombilla, but let's just call the starting end "Argentina."

Eventually your mate will become *lavado* and this is when you can pull out your bombilla, while carefully preserving the opposing mountain of mate and "switch hemispheres" by repositioning the bombilla in "New York," the northern hemisphere.

You'll create a new waterhole by firmly pushing the yerba to the opposite wall of the gourd. This, in effect, allows you to get at all the yerba reserves that were preserved in the other hemisphere, prolonging the cycle length of the mate.

Flooding the Mate

As you learned previously, the mountain of mate maintains the stable ecosystem of the yerba inside the gourd.

As you add water to your waterhole, you are extending the cycle life of the yerba by constantly keeping some of the yerba dry and unused as your reserve.

Once you're well into your liter, you can either practice hemisphere switching of the bombilla, or, you can "flood the mate" by indiscriminately pouring water over *all* the yerba and reincorporating the fresh reserves into the gourd.

Argentines are more prone to this sort of "flooding the mate," as I like to call it, than "hemisphere switching," which is more typical of Uruguayans with their significantly larger gourds and bombillas.

Unplugging the Bombilla

There are many reasons to unplug the bombilla from the mate, either partially or fully. The server needs to constantly maintain space around the bombilla, while preserving the precious mountain of mate. At times, it'll be necessary to totally remove the bombilla, replacing it in a superior position.

Unplugging the bombilla is good for removing cold pockets that form in your gourd, allowing you to achieve maximum heat retention with each fresh cycle. However, be careful, because the new cycle will tend to be relatively hotter – make sure to warn the Materos, if necessary.

If the bombilla becomes clogged, one of the best ways to correct the issue is to unplug (and run warm water through the bombilla) and reinsert.

Keeping your Mate Water Hot

It's a good idea to keep the cap on your thermos; if you're using an adjustable screw-on top, keep it tightened between cycles. This helps extend the heat of your water by preventing loss of steam.

Chapter 6

Mate Pairings

Mate with Sweets

Mate is bitter and cookies are sweet, so what better combination? When I'm in New York, there's nothing like stacking a pile of organic fig newtons alongside my mate. In Argentina, don't be surprised to see me munching on some *medialunas de manteca,* sweet croissants, hot off the racks from one of the many local bread shops, *panaderías,* peppered throughout the city.

Though I must admit, I usually drink mate *without* food. Mate is good enough to stand alone. But it's fun, now and then, to eat something sweet with mate, especially if I'm with friends. Those that like mate without sugar may enjoy something sweet with their yerba, to offset and balance the natural bitterness.

You can't go wrong with just about anything sweet. In Buenos Aires, *facturas* – an array of sweet croissants, to powdered cookies, to chocolate chip bread, to cream-filled pastries – are readily purchased and consumed in many a circles.

Pastry and Mate Pairings

Below are some ideas to get you started:

- *Toasted cinnamon raisin bagels with honey or butter*
- *Banana nut bread*
- *Blueberry bagel*
- *Waffels*
- *French toast*
- *Donuts*
- *Cereal bars*
- *Toasted bread with jelly*
- *Pancakes*
- *Vanilla waffers*
- *Pound cake*
- *Apple tart*

Mate and Cold Pizza

Today a friend and I drank several liters of mate and spoke for hours about life. She's from here and I'm from abroad, bridging the gap between continents and experiences.

"A" tells me how much she loves drinking mate with cold pizza. "You get yourself a pizza one afternoon, eat a few slices, then place the rest in the fridge overnight. The next day, for breakfast or lunch, make some mate and eat the cold pizza."

"Really?" I asked with amazement.

"Yeah, really!" she replied. "There's something about the taste of the cold sauce and cheese with a hot mate. It's so, so, so good."

"But are there many people who like this [in Argentina], or is it *just you*?" I questioned.

"No, no… plenty of people love this combination. You need to try it!"

Some months later, I tried cold pizza with mate and it didn't taste bad at all. The warm mate with the cold tomato sauce made for a unique flavor and texture.

A 2012 health article on yerba mate published in the newspaper *Clarín,* confirms the seemingly odd, but practiced combination of cold pizza and yerba:

> *Drinking yerba mate does a body well. The old axiom that from personal experience all Argentines know by heart now has a new scientific basis. Not only is it a great excuse to chat with friends, a faithful companion of savory biscuits or pizza fresh from the fridge, or an efficient homemade laxative…[1]*

Mate and Bizcochos

These pasty crackers come in two styles: salty and sweet. They're extremely doughy and greasy. The traditional Bizcocho (Don Satur variety) cracker is at the pinnacle of mate and food pairings. Ask any Argentine what sort of cracker or cookie is to be eaten with mate, and they'll undoubtedly proclaim "Bizcochos!" as if it were criminal not to have already known this eponymous tenet.

These hardy crackers are excellently paired with almost any sort of yerba, harmonizing your palate with buttery flavors mixing with the more bitter and smoky tones of the yerba.

Mate and Alcohol / Energy Drinks

In a taxi heading to the ferry on my way to Colonia, Uruguay, one animated and excited driver overheard me talking mate with my friend and started schooling me on the "ways of the Gaucho."

This brash and loud Argentine unreservedly told how "the true mate drinker is the Gaucho," and the "Gaucho wakes up in the cold morning, in the fields, after a long day of work, and begins his day with a few glasses of gin, then proceeds to mix mate with gin for energy, vitality, and the force to work another long day."

I've also heard of people mixing their mate with vodka and liquors. I can see how it would provide an initial rush of energy, as alcohol begins as a stimulant, then quickly folds into a depressant.

Together, the mixture of mate and alcohol doesn't make much sense, as mate clears the mind and alcohol usually muddles the mind (when drunk heavily). They are oppositional forces!

However, I can see how, if done right, some alcohol would benefit from the aid of mate in terms of a "mild drink." Perhaps a mate beer with a low alcohol content and a high injection of mate extract would be interesting.

I hear of a MateVeza, "a naturally caffeinated organic beer," already produced in the States; and then there's Club-Mate, originating from Germany—an energy drink loaded with mate extract and caffeine, highly popular in the computer programming and hacking community. There is also Mier, a relatively new mate beer made in Berlin by the Meta Mate Company.

Then there's Guayakí, the leading US mate company. With over twenty mate selections, the majority of their $13 million yearly sales comes from their bottled mate products

—including energy shots, mate drinks, and their latest entry, Sparkling Mate. Most of their mate is not pure yerba, but infused with a variety of fruits and herbs: mint, cranberry, grapefruit, lemon, raspberry, blackberry, honey, etc.

As mate becomes more accepted and known throughout the world, I'm sure that companies will incorporate it into their energy and alcoholic drinks; only time will tell. Nevertheless, nothing will ever trump a pure and simple traditional mate gourd and bombilla.

Less is more.

Mate and Cigars

Cigars and mate go together very well. If you're not a cigar smoker, then obviously the marriage won't make sense, but there's something about the strength of a nice, mature *(maduro)* cigar, coupled with a strong, Gaucho mate. Similar to a full-bodied red wine with a steak. I imagine the Gauchos did just that: smoke tobacco and share strong mates in the open country, around the fire.

Taking a few puffs of my cigar and a few sips of mate and I'm getting down

To business,
As I stare out my 8th floor in Buenos Aires.

Reflection. Contemplation. Meditation.

Cars interweaving streets.

An hour goes by and I'm still standing at the window,
As I have since a young child,

Now with my mate and cigar,

Alternating: mate and thermos on the ground after having a cycle, then some time to focus on my cigar, then back to picking up my mate and pouring a fresh one.

Heaven.
Smoky.
Inhale.
Exhale.
Relight.

Mate Pairings

Delight.
Sip.
Refill.
Chilllll....

People are the ants of the avenues.
Uruguay across the river.
Microcentro to my left.
Puerto Madero behind.

Chapter 7

Types of Yerba

Mate comes in various shapes, textures, tastes, and colors. The shape and texture – or composition – of the yerba is referred to as the cut. From broad leaves to an abundance of powder, each yerba has its own personality and style.

With Stems *(Con Palos)*
and Without Stems *(Sin Palos)*

Just as tobacco is cut differently, depending on the origin, leaf type, and preference of the grower and market demand, so is mate processed and classified into different cuts. Mate either comes with or without stems, known as *palos* (PAH-lows) in castellano.

Con Palos

The yerba includes chopped stems with the leaves and dust, making it a smoother and more balanced tasting yerba.

Sin Palos

The stems have been removed from this yerba and the pure leaf remains. This yerba is usually more robust and has more of a bite.

The Primary Mate Cuts

Gaucho Mate, or **Gaucho Cut**, is a very fine cut with plenty of powder, *(polvo)* and pulverized stems *(palos)* and leaves; this yerba is typically strong and full-bodied, with espresso and dark chocolate flavors, mostly drunk in Brazil and Uruguay. Such brands include: Canarias, Baldo Galaxy, Kraus Gaucho, Del Cebador, Mate Factor, Sara, etc.

> *Note: Keep in mind that Uruguay doesn't grow their own yerba, though several prominent mate companies are Uruguayan; their yerba is mostly grown in Brazil with a unique style that produces rich, robust, and malty taste profiles as seen in the country's flagship brand Canarias.*
>
> *These yerbas differ from the Brazilian yerbas (also grown in Brazil, but by local companies: Traditionally known as Chimarrão, pronounced "shim-a-HOW"),*

which typically are cut with an extremely fine, powdery grain, similar to Japanese matcha tea; it also includes, rather awkwardly, large stems and no leaves. A US-based company, Project Mate Bar, produces such Brazilian yerba.

A particular mate may be grown in a certain country, but it doesn't have to adhere to the typical cut of the country. As with Kraus Gaucho: A Gaucho Mate, but grown in Argentina. And with Mate Factor's Traditional mate: Grown in Brazil, but it's a clean cut yerba (no dust), not Gaucho.

Within Brazil, there are three sub-categories for classifying the mate's cut:

1. Moída Grossa: A coarse cut similar to Argentine mate. It contains leaves, stems, and medium grain powder.
2. Pura Folha: A cut that contains only leaves; no stems and powder.
3. Brazilian Traditional: Contains mostly medium grain powder, stems, and low content of leaves.

The most common cut is the *Argentine Cut*, which I classify as broad-cut leaves, light-to-medium-bodied strength, low amounts of powder, and large stems. Brands include: Mission, Nobleza Gaucha, Unión, Cruz de Malta, Kraus Orgánica, Amanda, Piporé, and Rosamonte.

The *Paraguayan Cut* is an interesting hybrid between the Argentine and Gaucho cuts: it contains plenty of fluffy powder as well as pulverized stems and leaves. This cut is light-to-medium-bodied. What makes this cut special is that, unlike a Gaucho cut, it contains stems; and unlike an Argentine cut, it contains an abundance of powder. Brands include: Ascension, Palo Alto, La Rubia, Selecta, and Pajarito.

Note: Apart from their unique sweet and sour tastes, Paraguayan yerbas are also aged longer – upwards of 3 years – creating blossoms of floral and subtle taste profiles. The Paraguayans seem to cut their yerba in a signature way that truly distinguishes the taste and characteristics from other cut philosophies.

The *Clean Cut* is an interesting cut found in North American yerbas. It's comprised of clean, slick appearing broad leaves; no stems; no powder.

The companies Aviva and Eco Teas are examples. Some think that removing the powder and stems makes for a superior yerba. It comes down to personal preference, really.

I absolutely love mate with *palos,* as long as the ratio between *palos, polvo,* and leaves is balanced (this doesn't apply so much to Gaucho mate). A mate without any *palos* and *polvo* is pretty boring; it lacks character, robustness, and the sort of viscous, syrupy consistency that gives roundness to the flavor.

Granted, the average North American mate drinker hasn't been as exposed to the wide varieties of mate ubiquitous to drinkers in Argentina, Uruguay, Paraguay, and Southern Brazil. (Remember, mate there is like coffee in the US. In the States, there are less than a dozen notable yerba mate brands: Guayakí, Circle of Drink, Eco Teas, Mate Factor, Aviva, Project Mate Bar, Oregon Yerba Mate, Nativa, and WyndHorse. Conversely, South America produces a few hundred brands.)

Guayakí, in business since 1996, is currently the largest supplier of mate beverages in the United States with roughly 60% of the market.[1] However, Eco Teas sells the most loose-leaf mate in the country.[2]

The North American mate market still seems trivial compared to the South American market, where mate is not only consumed by tens of millions, but remains an integral hallmark of the culture.

In that light, the American mate palate remains highly underdeveloped – not from a lack of yerba, as many brands can be purchased from online sources (yerbamateland.com) and health stores such as Trader Joe's and Whole Foods – but more from less awareness of mate.

Top brands in Argentina such as Taragüí and Rosamonte have never been experienced by the new mate drinker who's only acquainted with North American brands. I expect as mate continues to expand, not only geographically, but through cultural borders, more North Americans will have an impetus to broaden their yerba horizons.

I'm always delighted to receive messages from people following my work with mate, unashamedly confessing how they ordered three different types of yerba and how excited they are to try new brands. This gives me high hopes for mate in my country!

Yerba Characteristics

Gaucho Mate

Though many cuts appear and *are,* in fact, similar, there is a noticeable gap between Gaucho mates and the more common, Argentine mates.

Gaucho mates are very distinct in nature: the equivalent of what we'd refer to as "Cowboy Coffee" in the United States. "Gaucho" means "Cowboy." The Gaucho was the Cowboy of South America that roamed the *Pampas*—lands that spanned primarily between Argentina, Uruguay, and Brazil. Some Gauchos still roam these lands, tending to cattle, cultivating farmland, and raising horses.

The cut of the yerba plays a part not only in taste, but the overall environment – what I refer to as the "mate's ecosystem" – of how the yerba comes to life in the gourd.

Mate containing a lot of dust with little to no stems, found in Brazil and Uruguay, usually creates a pasty, cakey, and more viscous drinking experience. It's similar to matcha tea: a thick, talc-like traditional tea drunk in the Japanese tea ceremonies, now found in Western tea shops.

Galaxy and Canarias are traditional Gaucho cuts, producing malty and stout taste characteristics, with sweet hints of cinnamon, honey, and toasted bread. To compare these yerbas to the more traditional Argentine brands – since the taste, texture, and composition are so drastically different, and to suggest that one was better than another – would be akin to arguing that apples taste better than oranges: each person has their own preference, and the most weathered, polished Materos appreciate *both* styles.

Oftentimes, I'll drink the lighter, more green-teay Argentine cuts in the morning, then begin to drink the more dank, earthy, robust Gaucho cuts in the late afternoons leading to bedtime. Gaucho cuts seem to taste better in the winter—maybe because they remind us of hot chocolate on cold afternoons. Argentine cuts, more like crisp green tea, do well in the warmer, summer months.

That's the great thing about mate: like wine, there's room to experience different types of yerba, emerging from various origins and growing philosophies.

You may hear that you need a "special bombilla" to drink Gaucho mate, but I don't find that statement fully accurate. I've successfully drunk finely ground yerba with all the traditional bombillas offered. Yes, it is true that some bombillas permit more of that initial dust to enter your mouth within the first few cycles, but I've found that to be quite unavoidable with *any* bombilla.

Overall, the bombilla that I've found to perform the best— not only with Gaucho cuts, but with all, is the spoon bombilla, e.g. Katana Bombilla™. With its series of dotted holes as the filter, and its spoon-like shape, it fits snuggly below the patty-like wad of yerba that forms with powdery Gaucho cuts, while preventing minimal dust from entering the bombilla.

Argentine Mate

This is the most common style of yerba. The four major brands of Argentina: Amanda, Rosamonte, Nobleza Gaucha, and Taragüí, account for about 80% of the country's market.

Other brands such as: Mission, Unión, Cruz De Malta, Kraus Pionero, Jesper, Cachamate, La Eqsuina de Las Flores, Playadito, La Tranquera, Piporé, and La Vuelta are all solid representations of traditional Argentine yerbas: a healthy amount of stems, relatively low amounts of dust, broad-cut leaves, and a fluffy composition.

Though these yerbas share, more or less, the same cut (several are produced by the same company), that is not to say that they taste the same—most have their own unique flavor, ranging from soft (Nobleza Gaucha), to harsh and bitter (La Tranquera); to extremely watery-tasting (Playadito); woody (Jesper); smoky (Rosamonte); etc.

Paraguayan Mate

Paraguayan mates show hybrid-like properties in that they incorporate all the cut profiles: with a good amount of *polvo;* pulverized leaves and *palos;* medium-cut *palos;* and a distinguishing factor preventing it from being a Gaucho mate: the inclusion of medium-sized leaves and stems.

I love the molding that can be done with this yerba (and with Gauchos). You can use your bombilla as a carving tool, particularly if you're using a spoon bombilla, and shape the cakey yerba in any direction, maintaining a clean waterhole. You can't do this quite as easily with the less dense, fluffy nature of the Argentine yerbas, containing significantly less *polvo* (which acts as your mortar).

The Paraguayan yerbas are usually aged longer than their Argentine counterparts. Palo Alto is aged for 3 years before reaching the market. Pajarito, the most notable brand of Paraguay, is aged 2 years. Compare that with a brand like Mate Factor, shipping their yerba to market within 5 days of harvesting—the methods are like night and day.

These protean yerbas offer highly versatile, well-balanced tastes—kaleidoscopic swirls of smoked hickory, velvety dark chocolate, mild tobacco, and robust maltiness that's not over-the-top, but remaining smooth without losing its backbone.

Smoked (Barbacuá) and Unsmoked Mate

All mate undergoes a heating process, even if it's only through the wind and sun. Heating mate is essential to decrease the humidity of the leaves and help the flavors blossom. This is known as the blanching *(secado)*, or drying of each side of the leaves—traditionally done by fanning the mate branches *(ramas)* over an open flame.

As technology has advanced, companies now use rotating cylinders that quickly heats the mate between 20 to 30 seconds in 1100°F temperature. During this time the oxidation of the raw material stops, and the yerba loses 80% of its humidity—acquiring its characteristic aroma and color. The entire process is done within 24 hours of the harvest.[3] In some cases, yerba is dried through hot flash technology (no flames), as used by Eco Teas.

The yerba is then left to sit in a temperature controlled room to further decrease humidity. Then the mate is stored *(estacionamiento)* to cure – achieving optimal taste and texture – on average of 12 months.

During the drying process, some growers may smoke the yerba with various types of wood (sometimes with mate wood). Brands such as Rosamonte, La Merced, and others use this smoking, *barbacuá,* method. La Merced, one of the largest suppliers of *barbacuá* yerba, describes the process:

This variety of [smoked] mate takes it's name from the traditional drying process derived from the primitive techniques used by the Guaraní Indians. It consists of a long and delicate process by which the leaves are exposed to the heat of a coal fire for an entire day, imparting a refined robust and smoky flavor.[4]

Unsmoked mate *(sin humo),* as you can imagine, is yerba that hasn't undergone the additional process of smoke. The mate has a cleaner, more soft-spoken taste.

Organic Mate

Most yerbas aren't organic, or at least not *certified* organic. Though, some companies will state the yerba was grown "without the use of chemicals."

All major North American brands are USDA certified organic: Guayakí, Eco Teas, Mate Factor, and Aviva. These companies also practice Fair Trade, which ensures that all workers are fairly treated and are properly paid.

Certified organic mates include, but aren't limited to, these following South American brands: Kraus Orgánica, La Esquina de Las Flores, Pajarito Organica, La Rubia, Amanda Organica, Fede Rico, La Merced Organic, and Jerovia Orgánico.

The top Uruguayan brand, Canarias (grown in Brazil), states that their mate is 100% natural and grown without chemicals. This company is also the producer of Baldo, which appears to be the same yerba.

Mate with Herbs (Con Yuyos)

Some yerba comes blended with a variety of herbs, including: mint *(menta),* pennyroyal *(poleo),* lemon verbena *(cedrón),* and tulsi.

Lady's Breath is a mate blend with peppermint (*peperina/menta*) and spearmint. Its clean taste excellently contrasts the more bitter and stouter Argentine and Gaucho varieties.

Other brands include: Cachamate's Mixed Herbs, Eco Tea's Holy Mate, and CBSé's *Hierbas Serranas* (Mountain Herbs).

Shade Grown and Sun Grown Yerba

There are two principal environments for cultivating yerba: plantation method, exposed to the open sun; and shade grown, under the forest canopy. Each method influences the strength and taste of the mate.

Mate grown on a plantation, a method practiced by all major producers in Argentina, Brazil, and Paraguay, is exactly what you may expect: a clearing of a field into rows and columns of yerba—a monocrop.

This yerba, due to its unobscured exposure to the sun, is higher in tannins and caffeine, giving it a harsher, more bitter taste resulting in an increased effect of mate's energizing abilities.

Shade grown mate is, of course, more in harmony with Nature. The yerba is germinated in a greenhouse then dispersed throughout the forest floor to be grown in its natural habitat, communicating with other native species.

This yerba has a gentler tone and is generally smoother than sun grown. Though, Materos seeking that direct uplifting effect from mate will do better with sun grown.

Chapter 8

Mate and Health

Here, then, we have an ideal drink—one that is delightful to the taste, when once we have become accustomed to it; one that promotes digestion, gives immediate strength to the body and brain and acts soothingly upon the nervous system.

- WILLIAM MILL BUTTLER, YERBA MATÉ TEA:
THE HISTORY OF ITS EARLY DISCOVERY IN PARAGUAY

There're so many wonderful benefits to this plant. In fact, yerba mate is the plant that has the most nutrients of any plant grown on this Earth; any vegetable that you can eat, it has more nutrients in it …it's full of vitamins and it doesn't give you the jitters although it has the same amount of caffeine [as coffee], because it's nutrifying your cells.[1]

- DR. THERESA RAMSEY, CENTER FOR NATURAL HEALING

It is difficult to find a plant in any area of the world equal to Mate in nutritional value.

- PASTEUR INSTITUTE AND THE PARIS SCIENTIFIC SOCIETY

111

Mate's Abundance of Nutrients, Antioxidants, and Minerals

Traditionally, when Gauchos – South American Cowboys – would take long trips across the country, mate was literally their lifeline: due to the lack of vegetables and fruits – and the extremely high consumption of meat – mate became a vital source of nutrients, as well as a digestive aid, providing necessary vitamins and minerals otherwise unprovided.

In a modern comprehensive review of mate,[2] researchers Elvira and Heck showed mate to have an abundance of nutrients and minerals, with myriad beneficial effects on the body.

Primary benefits found include: cardiovascular improvement, central nervous system stimulation, cholesterol lowering properties, high antioxidant capacity to combat free radicals (dangerous molecules responsible for disease), anticancer, anti-mutagenic, antiviral, anti-inflammatory, anti-aging, and anti-obesity effects.

Below, in this section, I have outlined Elvira's principal health statements on mate:

Vitamins

Vitamins, essential nutrients derived from foods, are necessary for optimal health. Mate contains the following:

A, C, E, B1, B2, Niacin (B3), B5, B Complex, riboflavin, Vitamin C Complex, magnesium, calcium, iron, sodium, potassium, manganese, silicon, phosphorus, chlorophyll, choline, inositol, and pantothenic acid.

Polyphenols and Antioxidants

Polyphenols are compounds that work as antioxidants to protect cells from free radical damage. Mate has such a high concentration of polyphenols that "from the biological standpoint, [mate's] polyphenols act similarly as the body's 293 natural antioxidant enzymes and may prove to be potent supporters of [body's] systems."

Mate contains the following antioxidants:

Caffeic acid, caffeine, caffeoyl derivatives, caffeoylshikimic acid, chlorogenic acid, feruloylquinic acid, kaempferol, quercetin, quinic acid, rutin, and theobromine.

Mate was found to have higher antioxidant properties than tea, inhibiting more free radicals than both green and black varieties.

Minerals

Aluminum, chromium, copper, iron, manganese, nickel, potassium, and zinc.

Saponins

Anti-inflammatory and immune-boosting compounds, responsible for mate's bitter taste and foamy bubbles.

The saponins in mate were also found to be effective in decreasing lung inflammation associated with cigarettes.[3]

Biological Activity

Caffeine

Anti-carcinogenic, anti-obesity, antioxidant, antitumor, diuretic, energizer, stimulant, vasodilator.

Chlorogenic acid

Antioxidant, analgesic, anti-atherosclerotic (keeps the arteries clear of plaque buildup), antibacterial, anti-diabetic, anti-tumor, choleretic (stimulates liver health).

Chlorophyll

Antibacterial, anticancer.

Choline

Anti-diabetic, cholinergic (nerve health), lipotropic (enhances fat metabolism, preventing fat buildup).

Nicotinic acid

Choleretic, hypocholesterolemic (lowers cholesterol).

Pantothenic acid

Anti-allergic, anti-arthritic (helps prevent arthritis), anti-fatigue.

Rutin

Antioxidant, anti-tumor, anti-ulcer, vasodilator.

Tannin

Antioxidant, anti-tumor, anti-tumor-promoter, lipoxygenase-inhibitor, MAO-inhibitor[e] (anti-depressant).

Theobromine

Uplifts mood, diuretic, stimulant, myorelaxant (relaxes muscles).

Theophylline

Diuretic, choleretic, stimulant, vasodilator, myorelaxant.

Ursolic acid

Analgesic, antioxidant, antiperoxidant, antiarrhythmic (protects heart against irregular beating), anticancer, anti-alzheimer.

Mate's Broad Health Benefits

In Scutellá's, *El Mate, Bebida Nacional Argentina*, doctors and scientists speak highly of mate's health benefits.

The book devotes several pages of quotes from around the world attesting to mate's abundance of health properties. Here are some selected excerpts of their findings: [4]

- *Mate is used to treat dyspepsia.*
- *Among the usual drinks to increase vigor and force in the body, mate, without a doubt, is the first place to look.*
- *Mate activates digestion and helps the body assimilate nutrition.*
- *Mate is a general stimulant, but in particular, it activates the intellectual and physical faculties.*
- *Mate regulates the heart, nervous system, and muscular system.*
- *Like alcohol, mate excites the intellect, but in a more soothing and calming way.*
- *Mate is good for fatigue and boosting moral and wellbeing.*
- *If the body is lacking nutrition, mate restores homeostasis.*
- *Mate allows you to work long hours without eating.*

- *Mate acts as a natural laxative and diuretic.*
- *Unlike coffee, mate doesn't cause insomnia and doesn't agitate the nerves.*
- *Increases lucidity and clarity of mind.*
- *Good chlorophyll content.*

"Mateine" vs. Caffeine

In 1947, Argentine MD, Dr. Bernardo Houssay, Nobel Prize Winner in Physiology, stated "The active principal chemical of mate, commonly called mateína, [mateine] is an extraordinary stimulant that benefits the body."[5]

Whether "mateine" exists as a unique chemical or is being used colloquially to represent the combination of caffeine, theobromine, and theophylline, is no longer a question of scientific fact – as you will soon see that mateine is *not* a chemical, but a cultural term derived from – now-debunked – outdated research.

One Dr. Mowrey believes that mateine is a unique chemical *(not caffeine)*, claiming that mateine is a stereoisomer (a rearrangement of caffeine molecules, creating a new chemical) of caffeine:

Chemical assays on mate have traditionally looked for caffeine. In such tests mateine, being a simple stereoisomer of caffeine, would test positive. Until recently nobody has looked at the exact structure of the molecule—and, to my knowledge, nobody in the United States has ever made the attempt. Researchers at the Free Hygienic Institute of Hamburg, Germany, concluded that even if there were caffeine in mate, the amount would be so tiny that it would take 100 tea bags of mate in a six ounce cup of water to equal the caffeine in a six ounce serving of regular coffee. They make the rather astute observation that it is obvious that the active principle in yerba mate in not caffeine! But then, we know for sure it is not caffeine, for caffeine is not present at all.

Mateine has a unique pharmacology and it is unfair to compare it to caffeine...[6]

However, is it known that the caffeine molecule *lacks* a stereocenter, a linking point in a molecule making it possible to create a stereoisomer, in our case, mateine—negating any claim of mateine existing altogether.

Some companies will state that mate contains mateine with the backing of the study conducted by Dr. Jose Martin (as Mowrey quoted in *his* study), director of the National Institute of Technology in Paraguay. Though, when contacted by an investigator of the issue, the now ex-director, whose name is actually Jose Martino, said "there is no unique chemical structure for mateine and that yerba mate contains caffeine, just as coffee." [7]

Well known holistic health expert, Andrew Weil, contributes to the debate:

> *Some scientists contend the primary type of xanthine in maté is actually "mateine," a compound they say is chemically similar to caffeine but with slightly different effects. Some South American researchers claim that unlike caffeine, mateine induces sleep, and while it's a stimulant, doesn't trigger the jitteriness associated with caffeine. I don't agree with them.* [8]

When I was around the age of thirteen I started to drink coffee. Like a lot of children my age, we loved to purchase Starbucks Cappuccino cold drinks. When I was a little older, in high school, I begun drinking more traditional coffee, in a mug, before going to school, and after school, several times per day.

I loved the caffeine rush. As a chess player, I found the sharp cognitive boost in memory, analytical skills, and the ability to think faster, appealing. However, within a few years of drinking coffee, I started to have heart palpitations. Simply walking up a flight of stairs would send my heart into a tachycardia. I was drinking *too much* coffee. At my peak, probably over 1 liter per day.

The thing about coffee is that you can never get enough of it. The rush is addictive. The rapid uptake in cognition is something we seek out in the morning and is to be maintained throughout the day. *It's the corporate crack.*

I still drink coffee, but hardly these days. After five-years of drinking mate, my system, not surprisingly, *rejects* the hostile and clumsy nature of coffee. It's an aggressive drink. Perhaps this is why I've grossly decreased my alcohol intake in equal fashion.

The drinks that cloud my mind and *increase unconsciousness* seem to have less and less room in my life; I'm more interested in the drinks that *increase consciousness* and bring about clarity of body and thought.

I don't believe that the caffeine in mate works the same as it does in coffee. To even compare the caffeine levels in mate and coffee is dubious: 1 cup of coffee contains 85mg of caffeine, and mate around 78mg; however, mate is often shared in a group, not simply in a one-cup fashion like coffee.

A participant may conceivably intake 1000mg of caffeine during several servings of mates, (assuming spent mate was being replaced with fresh) whereas a person may have a single cup of coffee in the morning and one in the evening.

This observation is the clearest testament to mate's caffeine content working differently than the caffeine found in coffee: after one cup of coffee, your heart may begin to race with jitters soon to follow. After *several* cups of mate, most people feel *calmer*, clear minded, and ready to tackle the day.

What more evidence do we need? Mate soothes and excites and coffee *only* excites.

> *The things we call the parts in every living being are so inseparable from the whole that they may be understood only in the whole.*
> - GOETHE

The caffeine in mate is a part of an entirely different complex of intricately woven molecules that make mate what it is: mate. *Not coffee*. It's like taking a dab of white and mixing it with red and blue, then taking a dab of white and expecting the same results when mixing it with orange and yellow.

The caffeine in mate, with its brother and sister compounds, theophylline and theobromine, and myriad vitamins and proteins encompass something original in and of itself.

No wonder why so many people talk about mate "*not giving me the jitters.*" With years of steady mate drinking, I have never once experienced any jitters or jarring coffee-like effects.

Interestingly, mate has the dual ability to help you wake up as well as fall asleep. This may be a result of mate's adaptogenic properties, aided by a group of compounds called saponins, which help to holistically regulate the body.

I've asked a few Materos to share how mate affected them:

Mate helps me forget about my troubles and I feel more positive and creative. The physical effects of yerba mate give me a completely natural energy boost without being jittery or crashing. It just makes me feel alive.
- MATT BRITT

[Mate is] way more to me than coffee. Its effect on my mind is more balanced, steady, and relaxing. - MATTHIAS BRAUN

Yerba mate is an elixir of life and mental clarity. It picks me up when I am down. Clears my mind's eye when it is blurred. After every infusion, I feel at peace. It is as if an unseen force connects everything. - JASON KING

Mate's Safety and Supposed Cancer Causing Effects

Yerba Mate has been consumed for centuries but it has only been scientifically studied in the last two decades. The growing worldwide interest in mate has made it paramount that research on this herbal tea continues, as it has shown extraordinary possibilities not only as a consumer beverage but also in the nutraceutical industry.

In regard to carcinogenesis, the most recent information suggests that the association between mate consumption and the occurrence of cancer may not be due to raw mate itself but to contaminants that may be present in processed mate.

The high temperature at which mate tea is consumed may also play a role. Therefore, post-harvest technologies need to be improved—especially the drying process needs to be optimized to completely eliminate contaminants. Additionally, good quality control, including thorough analytical testing, becomes imperative to insure its safety.

- ELVIRA DE MEJIA, JOURNAL OF FOOD AND SCIENCE, 2007

Some will ask, "what have I heard about mate causing cancer?"[9-10] And to those, inconclusive studies, there have been just as many, *if not more*, showing mate's power to actually *kill* certain types of cancer.[11]

Every food, if the scientist looks closely enough, can be said to cause cancer in some capacity. Cancer is the second leading cause of death in America. Even with the studies supporting mate's cancer-fighting properties, so few people drink it. Like any new herb, that's expected. More worrisome are the genetically modified organisms, nitrate-packed hot dogs, and glued-together meat.[12] And we worry about *mate?* A plant that's been vetted and consumed by ancient tribes for thousands of years.

Granted, mate is still the new kid on the block (in the US). Critical inspection is warranted, as with every food product. With far less scientific attention than green tea and coffee, whatever few reports that are published, unduly fall under more critical inspection.

With only several years of renewed pharmacological interest into mate's compounds and effects, it remains, more or less, an unknown entity in the States—looked at with suspicion and caution. I estimate a few hundred–thousand people, at most, drink mate daily in North America. There are currently no statistics on the exact amount.

In a recent review on the health effects of mate, published in the *Journal of Ethnopharmacology,* Bracesco took a defending position that mate does not cause cancer or abnormal cell production:

> *A review on the evidence implicating ilex paraguariensis heavy consumption with some neoplasias [abnormal cell production; i.e., cancer] show data that are inconclusive but indicate that contamination with alkylating agents during the drying process of the leaves should be avoided. On the other hand, several new studies confirm the antimutagenic effects of ilex paraguariensis in different models, from DNA double breaks in cell culture models to mice studies.*[13]

Not to totally discredit any of these reports showing mate's relation to increasing the potentiality of cancer – as I'm sure they're valid within the exact framing, or controls, of their respective experiments, and perhaps not taking into account other unknown and innumerable variables that are inevitably excluded in any given controlled experiment – but I believe the mounting scientific, and potentially more credible, *anecdotal evidence,* derived from centuries of consumption, are obvious: mate is a healthy herb to consume, *for most people.* Each intelligent person should do their own due diligence, not take the word of any authority – or even the *Guaraní* – outright.

The FDA, Food and Drug Administration, the governing body that determines the safety of food, has given mate a GRAS, Generally Recognized As Safe to consume, classification.[14]

Colon Cancer

In 2011 a study that brought mate attention was its success in destroying colon cancer cells in vitro (in glass). The study showed that chemicals derived from mate's caffeine were responsible for the breakdown of cancer DNA, resulting in its destruction. The conclusion of the study, conducted by Elvira de Mejia, Associate Professor at University of Illinois, Food Chemistry And Food Toxicology, was as follows:

> *The results suggest that diCQAs [caffeoylquinic acid] in yerba mate could be potential anti-cancer agents and could mitigate other diseases also associated with inflammation.*[15]

126

Oxidative Stress Reduction

Argentine researchers from CONICET, Institute of Chemistry and Drug Metabolism (Iquimefa), as reported in the newspaper *Clarín*,[16] as well as published in *Phytotherapy Research Journal*, have found mate to help prevent a process called oxidative stress, which, while occurring, the body's biological ability to react against disease is greatly diminished.

Mate contains a high amount of compounds called polyphenols, which have antioxidant properties. Antioxidants are responsible for neutralizing harmful, disease causing molecules known as free radicals.

The scientists have found that the antioxidant properties of mate aid red blood cells by protecting their membranes. When the body suffers from red blood cell destruction, a person may become anemic. Drinking up to a liter of mate per day may help prevent this from happening.

Moreover, oxidative stress is associated with a slew of diseases such as: "diabetes, Alzheimer's, Parkinson's, metabolic syndrome, and a combination of factors such as obesity, hypertension and elevated cholesterol and blood lipids, among others that increase the likelihood of cardiovascular disease or diabetes."

With Argentina drinking 6.2 kilos per capita and the mate-frenzied Uruguay drinking 9.4,[17] they are well ahead of the mate health phenomena. Hopefully North Americans will catch-on and catch-up, as our health may depend on it.

Mate and Osteoporosis

In a four-year study by the University of Cuyo (Mendoza, Argentina), 146 postmenopausal women who drunk at least 1 liter of mate a day were compared with 146 non-drinkers.

The results, which were published in the January 2012 issue of *Bone,*[18] the official journal of the International Bone and Mineral Society, showed a 9.7% higher bone density of the lower back and a 6.2% higher bone density in the hip region. "Yerba Mate consumption and body mass index were positively associated with bone mineral density."

The study suggests that daily consumption of at least 1 liter, the size of a typical thermos, may be helpful in the prevention of osteoporosis—especially for postmenopausal women.

Mate and Cholesterol

Elvira de Mejia, perhaps the foremost yerba mate researcher in the world, showed that mate improved heart health by lowering cholesterol. Her findings were published in the 2007 edition of *Planta Medica*.

> *Blood levels of the cardio-protective enzyme paraoxonase-1 were measured before and after healthy volunteers consumed either 0.5 liters of mate tea, milk, or coffee. Activity of the enzyme increased an average of 10 percent for mate tea drinkers compared to the other drinks.*[19]

Another study that sought to "verify the effect of mate consumption on lipid and lipoprotein levels on humans,"[20] showed that after 20 days of drinking mate, LDL, or bad cholesterol, was reduced by 8.1%; after 40 days, a reduction of 8.6%.

It also showed mate to have a synergistic effect with statins, cholesterol lowering drugs, taken by the participants. It was concluded that mate "may reduce the risk of cardiovascular disease."

Mate and Obesity

In 2009 a study, published in *Obesity,* mice fed mate lost weight. Levels of cholesterol, triglycerides, and glucose normalized. Researchers concluded that mate contained powerful anti-obesity properties:

> *In conclusion, our data shows that yerba mate extract has potent antiobesity activity in vivo. Additionally, we observed that the treatment had a modulatory effect on the expression of several genes related to obesity.*[21]

Mate and Diabetes

In a study involving 29 people with type-2 diabetes and 29 with pre-diabetes, three groups were created to evaluate the effects yerba mate had on the disease.

One group received 1 liter of mate per day, another went on a special diet, and the third had a combination of diet and mate.

After 60 days of evaluation, the type-2 diabetes subjects that received only mate showed signification reductions in LDL cholesterol, fasting glucose, and glycated hemoglobin.

The pre-diabetes subjects that coupled mate with

dietary change also showed positive results, though not as substantial as the first group, with lowered triglycerides and LDL cholesterol.

Published in *The Journal of American College of Nutrition*,[22] researchers concluded "Mate tea consumption improved the glycemic control and lipid profile of T2DM (diabetes mellitus type-2) subjects, and mate tea consumption combined with nutritional intervention was highly effective in decreasing serum lipid parameters of pre-diabetes individuals, which may reduce their risk of developing coronary disease."

Chapter 9

The Mate Harvest

Farms produce their mate in different ways, so it's impossible to give a uniform method of production, as there are too many philosophies and techniques on how mate should be cut, dried, smoked, etc.

Below, you will find the *generally practiced* method of mate production, from the greenhouse *(vivero),* to the bagging of the yerba *(envasado).*

Greenhouse *(Vivero)*

Mate seeds are germinated and cared for in a greenhouse up to 8 months. The plants are then transplanted to the field or forest and allowed to mature from 2 to 5 years before the first harvest.

The Harvest *(Consecha)*

The mature plants are now ready to be cut. Using a machete or hand saw, selected branches are cut from the tree. In some cases, on large farms, machines do the cutting. Plants are allowed a recovery period of up to 3 years before being cut again.

During the months of May through October, when the plants are in the process of rapid growth and high leaf production, the harvesting takes place.

Separation *(Quiebra)*

Taraferos, mate harvesters, eliminate unwanted branches and debris, keeping the best leaves. The selected yerba is spread, bundled, and tied into burlap bags called *ponchadas.* These bags are loaded onto trucks or carried on the backs of the harvesters for further processing.

The Drying Process *(Elaboración)*

Heating of the yerba leaves (Sapecado)

Drying of the yerba begins by rapidly flaming the sides of the leaves for 20–30 seconds at around 1112°F, expelling the water from the plant and destroying the enzymes that prevent oxidation of the tannins, preserving its green color. During this heating process, mate develops its characteristic flavors which are attributed to the oils in the leaf.[1]

Traditionally this is done by hand, over an open flame, but most companies now use large cylinders that quickly rotate the yerba through heat, without actual flame contact. Some companies, like Eco Teas, use a hot flash system to prevent a smoky flavor of the yerba. During this process, the leaves lose about 20% weight through dehydration.[2]

Drying (El Secado)

Within 24 hours of the heating, the leaves must undergo a drying period to further remove the humidity, down to 2–4%. The leaves are placed in a temperature controlled room, between 176 and 194°F, for 12–24 hours.

Processing (El Canchado) and Storage (Estancionamiento)

Now the mate undergoes a coarse shredding through a mill, then bagged, using natural fiber materials and stored for a minimum of 8 months—in some cases, 2–3 years as found with Paraguayan yerbas (Pajarito and Palo Alto).

The mate is stored in temperature controlled rooms where ventilation and oxygen levels are monitored to allow the yerba to unfold and develop its characteristic flavors and smells and colors. This storage process is a distinguishing factor throughout mate companies, backed by different processing philosophies.

Many traditional Brazilian mate producers will skip this process entirely, foil-sealing and shipping their mate within a week of harvest, resulting in a retained green and grassy flavor that's tasty, but short-lived.

Conversely, Paraguayan producers will allow their yerba to slowly age and develop, like a fine wine or whisky, resulting in a highly sophisticated and kaleidoscopic array of subtle tastes and aromas, not too unlike a high grade green or black tea from China that's been pressed into bricks and allowed to age for a substantial time.

Milling the Yerba (Molienda)

Now the yerba goes through various stages of further crushing, shaking, and separation to remove unwanted materials, large twigs, and undrinkable debris.

The yerba is classified into various cuts and varieties, such as: with stems *(con palos)* and without stems *(sin palos)*. Depending on the cut and type of yerba, the amount of dust and pulverized fibers *(polvo)* is determined to be included or excluded in the proportion of leaves and twigs, resulting in the final cut. Refer to page 98 to learn about the primary cuts of mate.

This final process greatly determines the taste of the yerba. Mate with plenty of stems is usually smoother and slightly sweeter; mate without stems and containing a lot of powder, is bolder and more robust. This is akin to sweet white wine (chardonnay) and full body red wine (malbec).

Packaging (Envasado)

The yerba is then bagged in food-grade paper or tin packaging and shipped to market, ending the production: from seedling to store shelves to your gourd.

Conclusion

A Mate and Love

By Lalo Mir

Mate isn't a drink…Okay, fine. It's a liquid that you consume.
But it's not a drink. Nobody drinks mate when they're thirsty.
It's more of a habit, like itching.

Mate is the exact opposite of television: it makes you want to speak with someone, and makes you think when you're alone.

When someone comes to your house, the first thing said is "hey" and the second is "want to drink mate?"

That happens in all homes.

In those of the rich and those of the poor.
Between chatty and gossipy women as well as serious and immature men.

Conclusion

Between the old and the young, while studying or playing.
It's the only thing that's shared between parents and children
without arguing or blaming each other for something.
Democrats and Republicans pour mate without question.
In summer and winter.
It's the only thing in common between victims and killers.
The good and the bad.

When you have a child, you give him mate when he starts
walking. Just add a little sugar and they'll feel grown. You'll
feel very proud when your little boy starts drinking mate.

It opens the heart.

After the years pass, they'll choose whether to drink it bitter,
sweet, hot, cold, with orange peels, with herbs, or with some
lemon.

When you meet someone for the first time, you drink mate.
If you aren't sure how they take it, you may ask: "sweet or
bitter?"
And they'll respond: "However *you* drink it."

Keyboards are full of yerba.

Mate is the only thing that all homes have at all times. *Always.*

With inflation; when there's no food; when there's military rule; with democracy; with whatever sickness or hardship we're facing.

And if one day there's no mate, you just ask your neighbor for some.

Mate doesn't refuse anyone.

The decision to stop being a child and start being a man occurs on one particular day. Not when you start wearing large pants, get circumcised, go to college, or move out. We become adults the day we begin drinking mate for the first time, *alone.*

It's not by chance. It's not just "whatever".

The day that a child puts the kettle on the stove and drinks mate for the first time alone, in that moment, he discovers his soul. The simple mate is nothing more or nothing less than a demonstration of values.

In solidarity we'll put up with mate when it becomes watery, because the conversation is so good.

In respect for the time to talk and listen—you talk while the other drinks, and vice versa.

And in all sincerity, finally say: *"Enough! Change the yerba!"*

Now the time for friendship is over.
It's the sensitivity of the boiling water.
It's friendly to ask, stupidly, "The water is hot, right?"
It's in modesty one pours a great mate.
It's the generosity of giving in the end.
It's the hospitality of the invitation.
It's the righteousness shared between each other.
It's the obligation of saying "thank you" at least once a day.
It's the ethical, honest, and loyal unpretentiousness found in sharing.

You feel included.
Now you know, a mate is not just a mate….

Translated by Dave Mate
Salud!

Mate Glossary

– A –

Algarrobo

A common Argentine wood. "Carob" in English. Produces light, reddish-brown gourds.

Amargo

"Mate Amargo" or "Amargo" means mate with no additives: sugar, agave, lemon, etc. It's pure yerba mate. This allows you to appreciate the natural bitter and sweet flavors. Preferred by Uruguayans.

– B –

Bombilla (bom-BEE-yah)

Metal filtered straw used to drink mate from a gourd.

– C –

Canchada

Process of coarsely grinding mate before it's stored for aging.

Cebador

The person who prepares and serves the mate. Each time someone is finished drinking, in a traditional circle, the gourd is returned to the Cebador for more water, then he or she passes the gourd to the next person (to his or her right).

Cimarrone *(sim-mah-RONE)*

Simple mate without sugar or additives. See "Amargo." In Brazil, it's called Chimarrão (shim-a-HOW).

Circle

The mate circle, or Circle, is at the center of the mate experience. The Circle is the symbol of mate, whether it's the single Matero (passionate mate drinker) or a group of Materos coming together to share.

Cycle

Term used to express the duration for the mate to become *lavado* (tasteless). It also means the "turn" of the drinker; for instance, the server will take the first two cycles to test the mate's quality and temperature before passing the mate to his right. Additionally, a cycle can refer to one complete rotation of the mate around a Circle; for example "let's have one more cycle before we go out."

– D –

Despalada *(sin palos)*

Mate without stems.

Dulce

"Mate Dulce" is yerba prepared with sugar or any sweet additive.

Dummy Mate

Name given to the first one or two mates drunk by the server to ensure quality.

Dummy Water

Non-heated water added to the gourd before heated water, helping to protect the mate from being burned and preserving the vital nutrients.

– G –

Gaucho

"Gaucho Mate" is yerba with plenty of powder and no stems. It's equivalent to "Cowboy Coffee" in the United States. Usually strong and full-bodied, with intense espresso flavors. Typical of Southern Brazil and Uruguay. Canarias, Galaxy and Del Cebador are examples. Gaucho is the term for Cowboy in South America.

Gourd

Hollowed and dried calabash (in squash family) used to drink mate. Also called a "mate." Wood, glass, and other materials are also used for gourds.

Gracias

Traditionally in Argentina and Uruguay, you say *gracias* when you no longer want to drink mate.

Green-teaing

The transition phase of a strong, well-balanced mate, entering into a watery, green-tea-like taste. Some drinkers absolutely love this transition and others meet it with rage: "the yerba is lavado!...change it!" Depending on the yerba, the teaing phase is quite pleasant—especially if you like tea.

– H –

Hemisphere Switching

Repositioning the bombilla from the initial side of the gourd to the opposing side, allowing you to extend the cycle of the mate by using the dry yerba that you maintained in the gourd (mountain of mate).

– L –

Lavado (lah-VAH-dough)

Yerba that no longer has taste. It's now time for the Cebador to make a fresh mate with entirely new yerba.

Long Cycle

Yerba that keeps its taste up to ¾ to 1 liter of water (standard thermos). Canarias and Mission are good examples of long cycle mates.

Matejuana

The experience of drinking mate while smoking marijuana. The combination may create powerful medicinal effects.

Matero/a

The true Mate Drinker that has a deep-rooted relationship beyond the yerba. Mate is a *way of life* for the Matero/a.

Mateware

Any tool used to drink, prepare, or store mate: bombillas, gourds, kettles, tins, etc.

Mate Cocido (co-SEE-dough)

This refers to mate that's bagged and prepared in the same fashion as green or black tea, in a mug. It's becoming increasingly popular in Argentina as well as the United States, with brands such as Guayakí, Circle of Drink, and Eco Teas offering varieties.

Mate Molding

Powdery yerba such as Gaucho and Paraguayan cuts give you the ability to mold the yerba inside the gourd, assisting with bombilla placement. The high amount of powder gives the yerba a pasty consistency, which any skilled Matero can use to their advantage when preparing mate and keeping the waterhole clear.

Mate Yuyos *(SHOE-shows)*
Argentine term describing mate containing any additional herbs, such as: peppermint, cilantro, mint, chamomile, etc.

– P –

Palos
Small chopped twigs of the mate plant included in the yerba, offering a sweeter and smoother taste. The twigs contain the highest amount of theobromine: a compound that helps you feel happy and relaxed.

Polvo
The dust (made from pulverized stems and leaves) that's added to most mate cuts—some companies remove it, i.e. Mate Factor and Eco Teas. Generally, dust is important because it gives the mate a strong, well-balanced taste. It helps hold the mate together and increases the cycle.

Ponchada *(also "emponchadas")*
Directly after the mate is harvested, it is piled onto a strong cloth and tied, usually in 100 kilo parcels; this bundle is called a *ponchada*.

Palo Rating System (PRS)
A 25-point rating system between 5 categories, determining: Cut, Body/

Texture/Taste, Nose, Finish, and Cycle. The average is the result is the mate's grade. Some yerbas may have a great cycle, but lack taste or have a bad cut, and vice versa; the system was designed to judge the *overall* experience of the mate.

Palo Santo – "Holy Stick"
A highly dense wood found on the Argentina-Paraguay-Boliva border used to make wooden gourds. It has a sweet and smokey scent, often imparting pine-like flavors to the yerba. The resin is said to have skin healing properties. The scientific name is *Bulnesia sarmientoi.*

– S –

Sapecado (sah-pay-CAH-dough)
The production of the yerba is now beginning; bags of the bundled leaves and stems are untied and the yerba is sorted out by a *Sapecador.*

Short Cycle
Mates with a short cycle become lavado quickly, usually within the first ¼ to ½ of the thermos. Mate Factor, Playadito, and Unión Suave are good examples.

Sin Palos
Mate without twigs.

Tapado (tah-PAH-dough)

When the bombilla becomes clogged it's *tapado.*

Tareferos (tah-REY-farrows)

Workers that harvest yerba mate.

NOTES

Introduction

1. William Mill Butler, *Yerba Maté Tea: The History of Its Early Discovery In Paraguay* (Philadelphia: The Yerba Maté Tea Company, 1900), 21.

2. David Goldenberg, MD. "The Beverage Maté: A Risk Factor for Cancer of the Head and Neck," *Head & Neck* 25, no. 7 (2003): 595–601.

3. Dora Loria. "Cancer and Yerba Mate Consumption: A Review of Possible Associations," *Rev Panam Salud Publica* 25, no. 6 (2009): 530-9.

4. Francisco N. Scutellá, *El Mate, Bebida Nacional Argentina* (Buenos Aires: Editorial Lancelot, 2006), 76.

5. Edward Albes, *Yerba Mate: The Tea of South America* (Washington: The Pan American Union, 1916), 14.

Chapter 1 - What is Mateology?

1. Evlira Gonzalez de Mejia. "Dicaffeoylquinic acids in Yerba mate (ilex paraguariensis St. Hilaire) Inhibit NF-κB Nucleus Translocation in Macrophages and Induce Apoptosis by Activating Caspases -8 and -3 in

Human Colon Cancer Cells," *Molecular Nutrition & Food Research* 55, no. 10 (2011): 1509–1522.

2. Guaraní Tribe, "Legends of the Guaraní," http://guayaki.com/mate/1894/Legends-of-Yerba-Mate-Origins.html (accessed May 15, 2012).

3. Mehmet Cengiz Oz. "Miracle Energy Drinks," *Dr. Oz Show Blog,* http://www.doctoroz.com/videos/oz-approved-miracle-drinks (accessed May 15, 2012).

Chapter 2 - Creative Clarity

1. Michael Talbot, *The Holographic Universe* (New York: Harper Perennial, 1991), 260.

2. Stephen Harrod Buhner, *The Secret Teachings of Plants* (Vermont: Bear & Company, 2004), 82.

3. Stephen LaBerge, Ph. D., *Exploring the World of Lucid Dreaming* (New York: Ballantine Books, 1990), 113.

4. Ibid., 206.

Chapter 3 - Mate Circles

1. Warren Peltier, *The Ancient Art of Tea*
(Vermont: Tuttle Publishing, 2011), 95.

2. Ibid., 96.

3. Hira Ratan Manek, "Sun Gazing Process," *Solar Healing Center,*
http://solarhealing.com/sungazing/ (accessed May 21, 2012).

Chapter 4 - Mateware

1. Scutellá, *El Mate, Bebida Nacional Argentina,* 111.

Chapter 5 - Preparing Mate

1. Peltier, *The Ancient Art of Tea,* 21.

2. Ibid., 33.

3. Masaru Emoto, *The Hidden Messages in Water*
(Oregon: Beyond Words Publishing, 2004), 45.

4. Peltier, *The Ancient Art of Tea,* 66.

Chapter 6 - Mate Pairings

1. Unknown Author, "More Benefits of Yerba Mate: A Discovery that Prevents the Loss of Red Blood Cells" *Clarín,* http://www.clarin.com/sociedad/beneficio-descubren-perdida-globulos-rojos_0_701329958.html (accessed May 16, 2012). [Original text in Spanish, translated by David Askaripour.]

Chapter 7 - Types of Yerba

1. [Interview] Matthew Askaripour, Stefan Schachter, "The True Story of How Eco Teas Came to Be, " *Circle of Drink,* http://circleofdrink.com/the-true-story-of-how-ecoteas-came-to-be-interview/ (accessed June 17, 2012).

2. Ibid.

3. Rosamonte, "Drying Process," http://www.rosamonte.com.ar/ [visit "Processing" section on website] (accessed June 17, 2012).

4. Las Marías, [Click on "Productos" then select "La Merced Barbacuá"] http://www.yerbalamerced.com.ar/ (accessed June 17, 2012).

Chapter 8 - Mate and Health

1. Dr. Theresa Ramsey, "Yerba Mate Tea—The Healthy and Delicious Coffee Alternative," *drramsey.com,* http://www.drramsey.com/articles/ yerba-mate-tea-the-healthy-and-delicious-coffee-alternative/ (accessed: July 7, 2012).

2. Elvira de De Mejia, "Yerba Mate Tea (Ilex paraguariensis): A Comprehensive Review on Chemistry, Health Implications, and Technological Considerations," *Journal of Food Science* 72, no. 9 (2007): R138–R151.

3. Bracesco, "Recent Advances on Ilex paraguariensis research: minireview," *Journal of Ethnopharmacology* 136, no. 3 (2011): 378–84.

4. Scutellá, *El Mate, Bebida Nacional Argentina,* 73–78. [Original text in Spanish, translated by David Askaripour.]

5. Ibid., 73. [Original text in Spanish, translated by David Askaripour.]

6. Daniel B. Mowery, Ph.D, "Does Yerba Mate Contain Caffeine or Mateine?" *Erowid.com,* December 2003, http://www.erowid.org/plants/ yerba_mate/yerba_mate_chemistry1.shtml (accessed: July 27, 2012).

7. Ibid., http://www.erowid.org/plants/yerba_mate/yerba_mate_chemistry1.shtml

8. Dr. Andrew Weil, MD, "Is Yerba Mate Tea Healthy?" *drweil.com,* May 7, 2012, http://www.drweil.com/drw/u/QAA401108/Is-Yerba-Mate-Tea-Healthy.html (accessed: July 27, 2012).

9. Ribeiro Pinto LF, T, "Mechanisms of Esophageal Cancer Development in Brazilians." *Mutation Research* 544, no. 2–3 (2003): 365–373.

10. Goldenberg D, "The Beverage Maté: A Risk Factor for Cancer of the Head and Neck." *Head & Neck* 25, no. 7 (2003): 595–601.

11. Mejia, "Dicaffeoylquinic acids in Yerba mate (Ilex paraguariensis St. Hilaire) Inhibit NF-κB Nucleus Translocation in Macrophages and Induce Apoptosis by activating caspases-8 and -3 in Human Colon Cancer Cells," 1509–1522.

12. Dan Noyes, " 'Meat Glue' Poses Health Risks for Consumers," *ABC7,* April 30, 2012, http://abclocal.go.com/kabc/story?section=news/consumer&id=8642900 (accessed May 17, 2012).

13. Bracesco, N, "Recent Advances on ilex Paraguariensis Research: Minireview," *Journal of Ethnopharmacology* 136, no. 3 (2011): 378–84.

14. FDA's GRAS List, "Botanicals Generally Recognized As Safe," *FDA,* http://www.ars-grin.gov/duke/syllabus/gras.htm (accessed July 1, 2012).

15. Mejia, "Dicaffeoylquinic acids in Yerba mate (Ilex paraguariensis St. Hilaire) Inhibit NF-κB Nucleus Translocation in Macrophages and Induce Apoptosis by activating caspases-8 and -3 in Human Colon Cancer Cells," 1509–1522.

16. Unknown Author, "Another Benefit of Yerba Mate: Preventing the Loss of Red Blood Cells," *Clarín,* May 16, 2012, http://www.clarin.com/sociedad/beneficio-descubren-perdida-globulos-rojos_0_701329958.html (accessed May 16, 2012). [Original text in Spanish, translated by David Askaripour.]

17. Ibid., *Clarín*

18. Andrea S. Conforti, "Yerba Mate (ilex paraguariensis) consumption is associated with higher bone mineral density in postmenopausal women," *Bone* 50, no. 1 (2012): 9–13.

19. University of Illinois at Urbana-Champaign, "Mate Tea Lowers Cholesterol," *ScienceDaily,* October 23, 2007, http://www.sciencedaily.com/releases/2007/10/071023163949.htm (accessed: July 7, 2012).

20. De Morais EC, "Consumption of Yerba Mate (ilex paraguariensis) Improves Serum Lipid Parameters in Healthy Dyslipidemic Subjects and Provides an Additional LDL-Cholesterol Reduction in Individuals on Statin Therapy," *Journal of Agriculture and Food Chemistry* 57, no.18 (2009): 8316–24.

21. Arçari DP, "Antiobesity Effects of Yerba Maté Extract (ilex paraguariensis) in High-fat Diet-induced Obese Mice," *Obesity* 17, no.12 (2009): 2127–33.

22. Klein GA, "Mate Tea (ilex paraguariensis) Improves Glycemic and Lipid Profiles of Type 2 Diabetes and Pre-diabetes Individuals: A Pilot Study," *The Journal of American College of Nutrition* 30, no.5 (2011): 320–32.

Chapter 9 - *The Mate Harvest*

1. Scutellá, El Mate, *Bebida Nacional Argentina,* 157.
[Original text in Spanish, translated by David Askaripour.]

2. Ibid., 158.

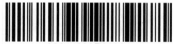

Made in the USA
Columbia, SC
24 October 2018